Full of it!

The shocking truth about gluten

(The brain – grain connection)

Dr Rodney Ford
MD MBBS FRACP

Foreword by Ron Harper

Is your brain being damaged by gluten grains?
The theory is that gluten can seriously affect your brain.
Are you or your family affected?

One -in-ten people are affected by gluten.
Are you the one? Find out!

Full of it!
The shocking truth about gluten
The brain – grain connection
Copyright 2006 RRS Global Ltd.
Author: Dr Rodney Ford

National Library of New Zealand Cataloguing-in-Publication Data
Ford, Rodney, 1949-
Full of it! : the shocking truth about gluten :
the brain-grain connection / Rodney Ford.
Includes bibliographical references.
ISBN 0-473-10407-5
1. Gluten—Health aspects—Popular works. 2. Food allergy.
3. Brain—Diseases—Popular works. 4. Celiac disease—Popular
works. 5. Gastrointestinal system—Diseases—Popular works.
I. Title.
616.975—dc 22

Published by RRS Global Ltd.
PO Box 25-360, Christchurch, New Zealand
www.doctorgluten.com
Printed by Tien Wah Press, Singapore

Jacket cover, art work and illustrations
by Liz Fazakarley of *Ford Design*.

Dedication

To yet more children and parents
who made this book possible.

"You can't wake a person
who is pretending to be asleep."

Navajo Proverb

Contents

Foreword by Ron Harper 7
About the author 13
Full of it! 15
The hypothesis 17
So what is new? 17

Gluten is it!

1. Gluten is it! 21
The problem with gluten 23
Gluten – invading your food 24
Problem symptoms have been officially "hidden" 26
How big is the problem? 29
More voices in the wilderness ? 30
Is it addictive? **32**
Gluteomorphines 33
Leaky Gut 35
The zonulin story 35
Leaky gut problems 37

2. What is gluten-sensitivity? 39
Gluten-sensitive problems 41
The ten target organs 42
You cannot tell unless you test 44
Coeliac disease history 45
The great masquerader 47
An explanation about blood tests 50
Small bowel biopsy 56
Is there an epidemic? 57

3. Gluten grains 59
Hunter Gatherers 60
The origins of grains 60
Grasses and grains 61
Bread and fast-foods 62
The food pyramid 63
Acidophilus 64
The shocking truth 64

Struck by it!

4. Your tummy brain **65**

What is your gut doing? 66
Oesophagus 67
Stomach 67
Small bowel 70
Large bowel 72
What is your brain doing? 74
How does your brain control your gut? 74
Autonomic nervous system 76
Gut feelings 80
Fight and flight 82

5. Gluten strikes your brain **83**

Symptom evidence 85
Gluten-brain connection reports 85
Neurological findings common 87
Poor response to gluten-free diets 87
Autoantibody damage 89
Gluten causing inflammation 90
Excitotoxins 91
Interfering with neurotransmitters 92

6. Headaches and migraines **93**

Medical evidence 94
Brain blood flow 95
People tell their stories 96

7. Nerve damage and stunted growth **99**

Neuropathy 99
Peripheral neuropathy 101
Motor neuropathy 101
Developmental delay 102
Autonomic neuropathy 105
Ataxia 106
Gluten-driven brain inflammation 108
Neurological dysfunction of unknown cause 109
Epilepsy 110

Stunted growth 111
Growth hormone suppression 111
The growth hormone evidence 112
Test all short children 114

8. Mood and behaviour 115
Lethargy, low energy 117
Angry 125
ADHD and learning problems 130
Autism 135
Depression 136
Psychiatric disorders 140

9. Tummy troubles 141
Gastro-intestinal motility disorder 143
Gastro-oesophageal reflux 144
Constipation and soiling 146
Diarrhoea and abdominal pain 152
Abdominal migraine 156

10. Got it! 157
Grains and your brains 158
Have you got it? 158
The critics 159
The criticisms 159
More answers to your questions 163
The gluten-sensitive patients 172
The storytellers 172
tTG results 173
IgG-gliadin results 174
IgA-gliadin results 175
Fantastic responses to gluten-free diets 176
Last words 177
Natalie's brown bread recipe 179

References 181

Foreword by Professor Ron Harper

This book can be seen as the missing link between gluten sensitivity and the brain. The breakthrough that this book makes is recognizing that it is not just the gut, but also the brain that is damaged by gluten.

For the last fifty years, the focus of gluten damage has been on the gut. Now, this book gives compelling evidence that the main injury that gluten causes lies in the brain and nervous system networks that control body functions. In short, gluten-sensitivity can be viewed as a neurological disease.

My entire professional life has been devoted to investigating the role which the brain plays in vital functions, such as breathing and cardiovascular control; it is impossible to find a body function not regulated by the brain and, of course, this includes gastro-intestinal functions.

So why would a brain physiologist be interested in gluten? The answer is that nearly all of the symptoms that are described in this book can be linked to disordered brain regulation. The mechanisms of injury appear to largely operate through damage to the autonomic nervous system, although other components of brain control, namely motor and thinking aspects, are also affected.

The autonomic nervous system is responsible for regulating the heart and blood vessel diameter, constriction of air passages in the lung, sweating and an extraordinary number of other body functions, including control of the nerves serving the gut.

Since the autonomic nervous system controls blood vessels diameter (and nearly all body tissue has blood delivered to it), substantial interference to the autonomic system would result in a wide range of symptoms – depending on where the damaged was seated.

Here, Dr Rodney Ford focuses on the entity of gluten-sensitivity rather than coeliac disease (also called gluten-sensitive enteropathy). The importance of this distinction is that detrimental effects of gluten are much more extensive than just the small intestine.

The critical concept of this book is that the body parts affected by gluten also rely on the brain to control their function, or supplies the blood to that part. Thus, in addition to the small bowel damage, gluten reactions can be associated with a number of brain-related brain dysfunctions (such as ADHD, autism, migraine, ataxia, tiredness and mental confusion).

In addition, brain nerve networks altered by association with reactions to gluten can create gastro-intestinal malfunctions which can be expressed as oesophagitis, reflux and heart burn, slow gastric emptying and bloating, and poor colon function with constipation and diarrhoea.

Neural control of the gut is largely performed by its own nervous system, with input from the autonomic nervous system, which in turn, receives direction from brain areas. The principal brain site in command of the autonomic nervous system is the hypothalamus, but the hypothalamus is itself controlled by many other brain areas, and autonomic nervous system outflow is limited by the cerebellum.

It is in the cerebellum that many of the damaging effects of gluten sensitivity impinge, eliciting such widespread effects, because the cerebellum modifies so many other body functions, including body movements and cognitive processes, in addition to autonomic outflow. The cerebellum exercises much of its control over the autonomic nervous system by influencing both the parasympathetic and sympathetic components of the autonomic nervous system.

The parasympathetic component of this autonomic system works principally through specialised nerves to the head, to the vagus nerve and through nerves at the lowest end of the spinal cord; the vagal and lower spinal cord nerves go to the body structures that regulate digestion and some portions of lung function. The sympathetic component innervates the heart, major muscles, and because it is responsible for constricting blood vessels, these nerves go everywhere where blood vessels go.

The principal target of gluten damage in the brain is the cerebellum. The cerebellum is a coordinating area; it compares the information felt by the body or intention to move with body motion. The cerebellum also coordinates input information with autonomic nervous system output, and injury can result in exaggerated blood pressure rises or falls, or excessive sweating, or constriction of the lung passages.

The cerebellum sends and receives nerve fibres from the frontal cortex of the brain, responsible for planning, and for suppressing distracting behaviour; two principal characteristics of attention deficit disorder. The reason why the cerebellum is such a target is because it receives input from long "climbing" fibres which are extremely sensitive to inflammatory or other influences, become too excited to such processes, and damages cerebellar cells through excitotoxic means.

It appears that gluten may elicit inflammatory processes which excites the climbing fibres, and damages cerebellar cells, resulting in the uncoordinated movement in patients sensitive to gluten, and the exaggerated autonomic patterns. The damage has been found in magnetic resonance imaging scans of the brain.

This newly discovered link between gluten and the brain explain a number of recent phenomena associated with the syndrome. Both ADHD and autism have increased over the last few decades, paralleling the increase in the fast food industry which mass-produces foods that are loaded with gluten. Gluten may be a major contributor to these rising numbers of neurological difficulties.

The "low carb" movement has also developed strongly over this time. The emphasis of these "low carb" diets is to reduce carbohydrates intake – especially white starches such as flour and breads. This change in diet is essentially a shift to a low-gluten diet; participants have unsuspectingly removed much of the gluten from their diet. Thus, many of the substantial benefits claimed by these diets may be attributed to the elimination of gluten.

Epidemiology studies show that more than 10% of the population show elevated IgG antibodies to gluten. This means that more than one in ten people are sensitised to gluten. The majority of these people are likely to suffer from some degree of brain dysfunction caused by their reaction to gluten. The particular body symptoms expressed depends on the site of injury to the brain induced by gluten.

The very high incidence of neurological disorders that are related to blood vessel regulation issues, including headaches, or directly related to cerebellar issues, such as attention deficit aspects, or disorders of movement or gait suggest that injury processes should be an object of attention. Any inflammatory process, such as found in response to sensitivity to gluten, should be suspect.

It seems to me that gluten is a strong candidate for causing widespread neurological damage. This book needs to be taken seriously and the ideas behind it researched in detail.

Ron Harper

Ronald M. Harper, Ph.D
Distinguished Professor of Neurobiology
David Geffen School of Medicine at UCLA
University of California at Los Angeles

"There is nothing permanent except change."

Heraclitus

About the author

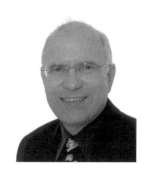

Dr Rodney Ford
Professor
MB BS MD FRACP MCCCH ASM

Dr Rodney Ford is a Paediatric Gastroenterologist, Allergist and Nutrition Consultant. He has been Associate Professor of Paediatrics at the Christchurch School of Medicine, University of Otago, New Zealand. People recognise that he has a worldwide reputation on adverse food reactions.

His major area of investigation has been the relationship between what you eat and what that food can subsequently do to your overall health. Rodney has been helping people with their nutritional problems and food reactions for more than twenty-five years.

Gluten-sensitivity (or intolerance) has been a focus of his interest over all of this time. He wants people to understand how food works in their body so that they can live a longer and more healthy life.

In his clinics he sees so many people who are eating the wrong types of food. By changing their eating patterns they can, at last, feel well again. He wants you to know about the meaning of every mouthful that you eat. He wants you to feel alive and be full of energy.

Increasing knowledge should create changes in thinking. There have been many changes on the perspective of coeliac disease over the last ten years, particularly with the advent of the blood tests. He wants you to understand the new thinking about gluten-sensitivity and its multiplicity of symptoms. He is now of the opinion that much of the damage that is caused by gluten is through its damage to the brain and nerve networks.

Rodney graduated with Honours from the University of New South Wales in 1974 (MB BS). He went on to study food allergy and intolerance problems in New Zealand, Australia and the United Kingdom; was admitted as Fellow of the Royal Australasian College of Physicians in Paediatrics (FRACP) in 1981; and was awarded his Doctorate of Medicine (MD) by the University of New South Wales in 1982 with his thesis titled: "Food Hypersensitivity in Children: diagnostic approaches to milk and egg hypersensitivity". It was a major work about the diagnosis of food allergy in children.

He runs a busy private allergy, gastroenterology and nutrition clinic. He has written over a hundred scientific papers including book chapters and books. This book is the fourth in a series of five books on gluten which puts forward his theory that symptoms from gluten reactions arise from brain and nerve damage. The five books in this gluten-sensitive series are:

o　　Are You Gluten-Sensitive? Your Questions Answered.
o　　Going Gluten-Free: How to Get Started.
o　　The Book for the Sick, Tired and Grumpy
　　　(Gluten-free KIDS).
o　　Full of it! The shocking truth about gluten
　　　(The brain-grain connection).
o　　The Gluten-Free Lunch Book.

Full of it!

This book is full of it! It is packed full of information that links gluten symptoms to brain and nerve damage. It is overflowing with information on gluten-sensitivity.

The title "Full of it!" is to capture the varied reasons for writing this book. It refers to our diets being full of gluten; to the world being full of gluten-sensitive people; to the medical practitioners who are so sceptical of adverse reactions to gluten; to the enthusiasm of people who are feeling vibrant again on a gluten-free diet; and to those who are brimming with hope that the problem of gluten has now been recognised.

The shocking truth

The shocking truth about gluten is that it is a food that is causing tremendous damage – but unrecognised. Gluten grains have become our staple diet. The quantity of gluten in our food has been steadily increasing. And official Health Policies endorse gluten grains as the foundation of our food pyramid.

But, all of the time gluten is sapping the energy and wellbeing of countless millions. And, as yet, the medical profession is turning a blind eye to gluten's wider problems whilst focusing all of their attention on the narrow problem of coeliac disease.

Can gluten damage your brain?

Searching questions usually provoke yet more questions. Answers can be hard to find. The big question that this book probes is: "Can gluten grains damage your brain?" I believe that the answer to this question is a resounding "Yes!". I have come to this conclusion by the abundant circumstantial evidence from my observations of my patients who are gluten-sensitive. I have pondered the next questions: "Why do they have such an array of symptoms from gluten?" "Why do they recover so quickly when gluten is removed?" And "Why do they deteriorate so rapidly when only tiny amounts of gluten are eaten?"

Over the last fifty years, there has been a slow evolution of the understanding about gluten toxicity. But each time that a new clinical investigation has been developed this new information is merely added on to the current theory.

Seldom is the whole concept re-examined. To this end, the focus of gluten has unwaveringly been on the small bowel. This is because coeliac disease is generally considered to be a gastro-intestinal disease, with some unexplained peripheral symptoms. Coeliac disease (also known as gluten-sensitive enteropathy) is defined as bowel damage caused by the toxicity of gluten in susceptible people. Recent population studies around the world show that it occurs in about one in every one hundred people.

I now challenge this narrow perspective. I have described the clinical features of a much wider condition – that of gluten-sensitivity. I have calculated that gluten-sensitivity affects about one-in-ten people. Others claim that it is even more common. In my opinion, gluten has now been recognized as the cause of a vast amount of chronic ill health.

The purpose of this book is to submit a hypothesis that provides a universal model of gluten-sensitivity. I believe that gluten-sensitivity is a brain and nerve network disease.

Read on and find out why.

The hypothesis

My hypothesis is as follows:

"The symptoms from gluten occur through
its action on the nervous system".

In other words, gluten-sensitivity is a brain condition. I propose that gluten can injure the nervous networks that control the gut's functions. This malfunction subsequently leads to all of the gut symptoms that have so well been described. In addition, gluten also directly affects the brain, which leads to the primary neurological symptoms that are so commonly seen with gluten-sensitivity.

Gluten can damage brains

What is new?

There are major new ideas in this book. They are based on circumstantial evidence. They give a unifying theory to the symptoms that are attributed to gluten toxicity.

1) A brain disease

I believe that gluten-sensitivity is mostly a neurological problem. A major contribution to this debate is the realisation that the brain has a central role in the expression of the symptoms that have until now been attributed to the local toxicity of gluten on the gut. Traditionally, gluten reactions have been thought to be from gluten directly damaging the gut tissue. However, all of these symptoms can be explained through their brain connections and the subsequent disordered feedback mechanisms.

2) A nerve disease

I propose that gluten-sensitivity is also a nerve disease. There is a gigantic network of nerves that controls every function that your gut is programmed to do. There are as many nerve cells in your gut as there are in your head! About 25 billion nerve cells. I call it your tummy brain (or gut brain). Your tummy brain can be directly damaged by gluten reactions. This is the cause of so many sore tummies and bowel troubles.

3) A wide spectrum of neurological manifestations

For decades, there have been reports of unexplained brain and nerve symptoms which are associated with coeliac disease. But, although these associations have been described, there has been no universal mechanism proposed. However, if gluten is regarded as a neurotoxin, then the explanation has been found. This toxicity may act through inflammatory mechanisms.

4) A very common disease

Reactions to gluten have been documented to be extremely common. About one-in-ten people (as ascertained by blood donor studies) have high levels of gluten antibodies in their blood. My clinical studies have arrived at this same high number of gluten-sensitive people. Dozens of population studies on coeliac disease have found that about one-in-one-hundred people are affected. However, I have demonstrated that coeliac disease comprises only a tenth of the gluten problem. I am unaware of any population studies that have documented the frequency of brain and nerve symptoms caused by gluten.

Why is this hypothesis so attractive?

This theory is attractive because it gives a unifying answer that explains the following conundrums associated with gluten:

o   The mechanism of the non-gut symptoms of coeliac disease

o   The behaviour disturbance side of gluten reactions

o   The psychiatric and personality disorders

o   The neurological symptoms

o   The autonomic system disturbances

o   Why such small amounts of gluten can cause such major reactions by the amplification effect of the nervous system.

How is this book structured?

In this book, I discuss the issues surrounding the new knowledge about gluten-sensitivity and present you with evidence. I believe this clearly indicates that brain and nerve networks are the primary targets of gluten toxicity. The structure of this book is based on putting forward a logical progression of the arguments which link gluten grains to your brain.

There are three parts to this book:

1) **Gluten is it!** – tells the story of the introduction of gluten grains into our diets and the problems that have stemmed from this agriculture development. You are introduced to gluten and the harm that it wreaks.

2) **Struck by it!** – explains how your brain is inextricably linked to your gut and everything that you do, day and night. It discloses the relationship between gluten and your brain. It documents the details from both medical and brain research

on how gluten can attack your brain. It also presents a series of narratives from my patients who had neurological dysfunction that can be attributed to gluten neurotoxicity. By reading their accounts, you can evaluate whether you or your family are likely to have any damage from gluten.

3) **Got it!** – do you have it? What should you do about it? How can you solve it? You will learn what to look out for and how to test for it. We then tell you what you can do to become cured. The clinical data from the patients who have told their stories has also been collated and summarised.

My hypothesis has been formed by my extensive dealings with gluten-sensitive children and adults, and from researching the medical literature. There is some repetition in this book to ensure that each chapter is complete. This is not a text book. It is a book expressing my opinions backed up by my patients. Relevant scientific references are given at the end. I thank all of the children, and the parents and my colleagues who have helped me so much on this fascinating and disturbing adventure.

You might ask, "Am I full of it?" Yes, I am full of excitement and hope for the future. So many people can be helped, if only this information can be widely distributed. I am full of ideas and full of enthusiasm. I hope that you are full of hope for your healthy and vibrant future.

The shocking truth is that so many people are being encouraged to eat gluten-foods that are steadily eroding their health and energy.

If you have any comments or questions we would love to hear from you through our webpage   www.doctorgluten.com

1. Gluten is it!

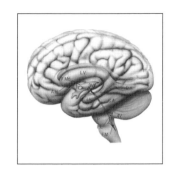

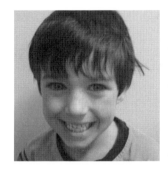

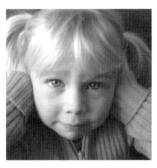

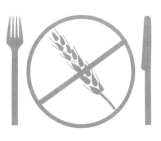

1. Gluten is it!

Gluten is it! Our diets are full of it. Our processed foods are full of it. You might be full of it. And the worst thing is that all of this gluten might be harming you, and your family.

Our food is full of it!

So, where does it (gluten) come from? The first thing you need to do is to learn more about the nature of gluten. Only then will you understand my reasoning. Gluten is a food protein which is relatively new to us in terms of our human long-term development.

The gluten grains come from the family of grasses. This family includes wheat, rye and barley. But gluten is also found in some of the other grass-like cereals of Spelt, Kamut and Triticale (a wheat-rye cross). These grains are also called golden grains. They all contain this gluten protein.

Gluten is found in wheat, rye and barley

Gluten is a substance made from protein. Gluten's function in these grass grains is to help with the protection and germination of the seed. It protects and nourishes the seed. It has been called a storage protein. It, therefore, needs to be resistant to biological breakdown while it is looking after the dormant and growing seed. It is a tough protein. This explains why our bodies have such difficulty in fully digesting it in our intestines.

One of the central problems of gluten is that it is an unusual protein. Your body does not handle it very well. Your gut cannot fully digest it. Thus fragments of gluten can be easily absorbed into your body in an unchanged form. Unfortunately, this can set up an immune reaction that can go on to damage your body parts – and I believe that this process can damage your brain.

Gluten is hard to digest

Gluten is a family name for a group of small proteins. The main family members include gliadin and glutenens. Gliadin is actually a group of proteins. It is the alcohol-soluble protein fraction of wheat. This collection of proteins contains the factor that is toxic to the gut for coeliac patients. Unfortunately, the toxicity of gliadin is not destroyed by the digestive enzymes that get produced by your stomach and pancreas.

The problem with gluten

People ask: "What is wrong with Gluten?" "How can an everyday food make me sick, tired and grumpy?" They say: "Surely a food cannot be so harmful!"

As I have already said, the big problem with gluten is this – it does not get digested properly in your gut. We humans are not equipped with sufficient enzymes to adequately digest this protein fraction completely. This undigested fragment can be harmful.

Gluten causes an immune reaction

For those millions of people who are susceptible, these short undigested protein chains (called peptides – see next section) get absorbed unchanged into your blood stream. This gluten invasion is immediately detected by your immune system. This undigested gluten (also called gliadin) is seen by your body as a foreign invader. Your body, therefore, mounts an immune response against it. This is the reaction that starts the damage. Gluten can also interfere with your other body systems. This has the potential to cause you a lot of damage.

Gluten creates a vicious cycle of damage

If you continue to eat gluten, then your immune mechanism will *continue* to react to the gluten. This reaction can get progressively stronger and stronger. This puts a vicious cycle in motion which, sadly, can lead to a vast spectrum of ill health. This wide range of symptoms, triggered by gluten, is now known as gluten-sensitivity. Coeliac disease (the gut damage caused by gluten) is a specific subset of these conditions.

Gluten – invading your food

Another big problem about gluten is that it is everywhere! You can find it in so many of your processed foods. In our wheat-based societies, most children, most adults, and most of the elderly consume large amounts of wheat-based products – at every meal, on every day, throughout their lives.

Gluten is everywhere

This means that they have *never* had any experience of being gluten-free. Therefore, it is impossible for them to know whether gluten could be causing them harm.

All of their lives, vast numbers of people have been feeling "under the weather", or have had minor symptoms that they have just put up with. The trouble is this: because they are perpetually unwell, they may not recognise that they are unwell. Being below par is their normal state of affairs. They know nothing else!

These people cannot recognise their lack of energy, or their tiredness or their uncomfortable tummy as a symptom – this is just "normal" for them. They have always had them. Sadly, these people do not know how fantastically well they would feel off gluten! Gluten-free might be their cure.

How do you know if you are normal?

Many minor (and sometimes major) symptoms are often put down to people's genetic make-up, or their intolerance to pain, or their poor immune health, or a degenerative illness, or being a hypochondriac, or being a trouble maker, or attention seeking. In the medical field these chronic lifetime ailments are usually fobbed off or ignored. In children they are dismissed as growing pains or a "phase" to outgrow.

However, a large proportion of all of these general ailments can be attributed to gluten-sensitivity. All of these people need a blood test. All such people need to be taken seriously. Most will respond to a gluten free diet.

So many people are "below par"

Here are some figures to give you some idea about the extent of the poor health that is experienced in our communities:

> 1 in 4 have asthma or hay fever or eczema.
> 1 in 10 children have learning difficulties.
> 1 in 10 children are labelled dyslexic or dyspraxic.
> 1 in 10 have constipation and/or diarrhoea.
> 1 in 10 have abdominal pain or irritable bowel.
> 1 in 15 children have been diagnosed as ADHD.
> 1 in 200 are diagnosed with Autism.

Many children often have several of these conditions.

Problem symptoms have been officially "hidden"

One of the most widely recommended books about common childhood problems is called "The Normal Child". This was written by Professor R. S. Illingworth and was first published in 1953. Its subtitle was "The development of the infant and young child, normal and abnormal." It has been revised a number of times, its tenth edition was in 1991. Over this time the subtitle has changed to "The normal child and some of his abnormalities (1967)" and "The normal child; some problems of the early years and their treatment (1987)."

Illingworth wrote this book to document the "normal symptoms" that he believed were experienced by "normal" healthy children. But what is not answered in his book is how he determined "who is normal". It is his viewpoint of symptoms in children who had no recognised organic disease. The symptoms that Illingworth describes as "normal" in childhood include: 10–15 % have recurrent abdominal pains; 10–15 % have headaches or migraines; 10 % have constipation or diarrhoea; 10 % have eczema; and about 5 % have limb pains or "growing pains". He classified these under the heading "miscellaneous behavioural problems".

Another author, John Apley, stated similar views in this same era. On recurrent abdominal pain he stated, "In 19 of every 20 cases theses pains go with emotional disturbances and are not due to organic diseases." He put these symptoms in a chapter called "Emotional and behavioural problems". In his list of "Emotionally determined bodily disturbances" he included: stunted growth; anorexia; constipation; irritable colon; sleep disorders; cyclical vomiting; and recurrent pains of the abdomen, head and limbs.

Coincidentally, these are the very same group of symptoms that I ascribe to gluten-sensitivity. Illingworth also describes these symptoms in the same proportions that I find in children who react to gluten. He speculated that these symptoms could be caused by abnormal responses of gut hormones. I think that he was right!

It is my argument that a "normal" child should not have *any* symptoms. In my opinion, the children who have symptoms that Illingworth has described as "normal" can now be diagnosed. They can now have a blood test and they can be found to be reacting to gluten. They can be put on a gluten-free diet and eventually they can be free of their persisting symptoms.

"The Normal Child" doctrine has been promulgated for fifty years. It has been a reference book for several generations of medical practitioners. It claims that over fifteen percent of "normal" children have chronic symptoms that have no foundation in any illness. This has had the effect of dismissing and ignoring these children's symptoms. The medical system has become blind to the suffering of these children and their parents.

Normal children should have no symptoms

The gluten-sensitive symptoms have been hidden in a cloak of "normality". This is a tragedy. Previously, because these symptoms could not be explained, they were categorized as "normal". With the advent of gluten blood tests, now history can be rewritten.

Autism

Some of the autism problem has been linked to gluten. Autism is becoming more and more common. The rising numbers of children diagnosed as autistic has been exhaustively investigated by Blaxill (2004). He says: "Increases in the reported prevalence of autism and autistic spectrum disorders in recent years have fuelled concern over possible environmental causes. The large increases in prevalence in both the United States and the United Kingdom cannot be explained by changes in diagnostic criteria or improvements in case ascertainment."

Autism is rife

"There are large recent increases in rates of autism and autistic spectrum disorders in both the U.S. and the U.K. Reported rates of autism in the United States increased from 3 per 10,000 children in the 1970s to 30 per 10,000 children in the 1990s, a 10-fold increase. In the United Kingdom, autism rates rose from 10 per 10,000 in the 1980s to roughly 30 per 10,000 in the 1990s. Reported rates for the full spectrum of autistic disorders rose from the 5 to 10 per 10,000 range to the 50 to 80 per 10,000 range in the two countries."

This means a diagnosis in 1 in 200 children. This is about a ten-fold increase.

How big is the problem?

The world seems to be full of it! A vast number of the patients that I see now turn out to have gluten-sensitivity. This is a huge problem.

One in ten have gluten-sensitivity

From my clinic data, I estimate that about 1 in 10 people in the general community are sensitive to gluten. Other researchers think that the gluten problem is even more common than this.

When you look at the chronically unwell group of people, then the problem is even more frightening. I calculate that about 1-in-3 who are chronically unwell might be gluten-sensitive. In other words, I suspect that up to a third of all chronic ailments can be attributed to their adverse reactions to gluten.

This has only become apparent over the last ten years since there have been reliable tests to detect gluten antibodies in the blood. The sad thing is that these tests are only being utilised by just a few medical practitioners. As yet, there is little medical belief in gluten-sensitivity. There is an absolutely enormous amount of ill health that could be eliminated in one swoop if gluten-sensitivity was taken as seriously as high blood pressure or high cholesterol levels.

You can't tell unless you test

Currently, all health professionals recognise that there is no way of determining how high your cholesterol level is except by doing a blood test. You have to have a blood test to measure your blood lipid levels. Likewise, there is no way of determining how high your blood pressure is without it being measured.

You have to have a blood pressure test to check for hypertension. Accordingly, exactly the same goes for gluten-sensitivity! You can't tell unless you test. But very few medical practitioners are willing to request these blood tests for gluten – so very few people are being diagnosed and treated.

Everybody should have a gluten blood test

When gluten antibodies are looked for, practitioners are finding huge numbers of people with gluten-sensitivity. But sadly, few tests are being done.

More voices in the wilderness

There are others who are sending out this urgent message about gluten-sensitivity. The recognition of gluten-sensitivity is gathering speed. There are other voices to listen to.

For his whole medical career, Kenneth Fine, gastroenterologist, USA, has been investigating people with diarrhoea . He noticed that most people who were gluten-sensitive did not have all of the necessary characteristics to make the diagnosis of coeliac disease. His population research has found high levels of gluten IgG-gliadin antibodies in the blood of 11% of the general American public.

One in ten people have high gluten antibodies

He has also looked for similar antibodies to gluten in the stool (faeces). His research has revealed that these antibodies are detected in the stool in as many as 35% of people who otherwise appeared to be normal people. He goes on to say that if high risk patient populations are tested (in other words, people with chronic symptoms), then the percentage of those with high gluten antibodies will exceed 50%.

Another two American clinicians, James Braly and Ron Hoggan (2002), in their book *Dangerous Grains*, state that gluten intolerance does not just affect a few people with coeliac disease, but as much as 3% of the population. They also estimate, "that between 10% and 15% of the US and Canadian populations have high anti-gliadin antibodies. This puts them at risk of conditions as varied as psoriasis, multiple sclerosis, jaundice, inflammatory bowel disease, and eczema."

The gluten evidence is overwhelming

Also, according to Dr Alessio Fasano (2003), who carried out his research at University of Maryland, USA, he states: "Worldwide, reactions to gluten 'outside of the intestine' are found 15 times more frequently than classic coeliac disease 'inside the intestine'".

Yet another researcher, Dr Ronald Hoffman (2004), was also impressed that IgG-gliadin antibodies, when looked for in the blood, were raised in 12% of the American public. In his clinic he says, "I find these antibodies positive in around 30% of my patients who have an array of challenging medical problems."

The overwhelming message is this: if you look for gluten-sensitivity in people who have chronic health problems, then you will find it! A third of these sufferers are intolerant to gluten. Moreover, when they go gluten-free they usually completely recover. I repeat – you can't tell if you don't test.

Is it addictive?

Is gluten addictive? Yes it is! The scope of the gluten problem just keeps on getting worse. Disturbingly, gluten has a morphine-like activity. This makes gluten addictive. It can behave in a similar way to morphine. As you may know, morphine is part of the wider group of addictive drugs that are called opiates. They include heroin and opium. These drugs are all similar substances which are used for either medical purposes for pain relief or by addicts to get their "high".

Gluten can give you a "high"

As humans, we actually produce a natural morphine substance in our brains – this chemical is called *endorphin*. These endorphins are released in our brains to give us a sense of pleasure. They are also released in our brain as part of our body's natural mechanism to help numb pain. They are addictive.

New research shows that gluten can generate some of these effects. Eating gluten can give you a real sense of pleasure. This fact can explain why some people seem to be addicted to wheat-based products. They are sometimes amusingly referred to as bread-o-holics.

Gluten can give a feeling of comfort

Eating cakes, dumplings, steamed puddings and big hunks of bread is often referred to as eating "comfort foods". For some people, this comfort is being derived from the morphine-like activities that the gluten is having in their brains. Yes, eating bread can be additictively pleasurable. Many people are desperate for their meal-time gluten fix. I call them bread-heads. The other side of the coin is that going on a gluten-free diet can lead to withdrawal effects. This is one of the reasons why a gluten-free diet is initially viewed by so many people as a horror story. Indeed, withdrawal effects from gluten on the first week of a gluten-free diet are not uncommon. It needs a real commitment to go onto a gluten-free diet.

Gluteomorphines

Here is the science behind this gluten addiction. The gluten protein is broken down in your body by gut enzymes into the smaller fragments called peptides. Some of these peptides are known as gluteomorphines: they have a morphine-like activity. The majority of people have the ability to further break down these peptides into even smaller units, the individual usable amino acids. These are harmless. These amino acids are then absorbed into your body and used to manufacture the many other proteins that your body needs.

Gluten fragments can act like morphine

But there is another group of people. Those who do not efficiently break down or eliminate these gluteomorphine peptides. This is probably due to these people having rather "leaky gut surfaces". This can be visualized like having bigger than normal "holes" in the intestinal membranes. This would then allow these hazardous peptides to get into your blood. Once these gluteomorphines are circulating in your bloodstream, they are able to seek out the specific morphine receptor sites in your brain (Knivsberg, 2002).

The biochemistry of exorphins that are derived from gluten is complicated. These exorphins belong to a class of biologically active short peptides. These peptides are very small. They are only about 4–8 amino acids long. They have this morphine-like, or opioid, activity. These peptides vary in their amino acid sequence. The following list gives some examples of these gluten exorphins:

Exorphin A5:	Gly-Tyr-Tyr-Pro-Thr
Exorphin B5:	Tyr-Gly-Gly-Trp-Leu
Exorphin C:	Tyr-Pro-Ile-Ser-Leu
Gliadorphin:	Tyr-Pro-Gln-Pro-Gln-Pro-Phe

In this table, the letters stand for individual amino acids
Tyr = Tyrosine
Gly = Glycine
Pro = Proline
Thr = Threonine
Trp = tryptophan
Leu = leucine
Ile = Isoleucine
Ser = Serine
Gln = Glutamine
Phe = Phenylalanine

These intact peptides can be absorbed from the small bowel. They are then transported by the blood stream and they eventually reach your brain. In most people, these peptides are rapidly broken down in the blood. Only tiny amounts of such peptides are eventually found in the urine (Marti, 2005). But, some people are more affected by these peptides than others. This problem is made worse by a leaky gut.

Gluten affects the brain

"Leaky Gut"

There is now good evidence that people who develop the condition coeliac disease have what is termed a "leaky gut". The medical term for this is "increased intestinal mucosa permeability". This means that the skin (mucosa) of the intestine lets through more of the intestinal fluids and chemical substances into your body. This is because the joins between the cells in the gut mucosa are not quite as tight as in other people who do not have such a leaky gut. The diagram illustrates this. The top row of cells are normal ...

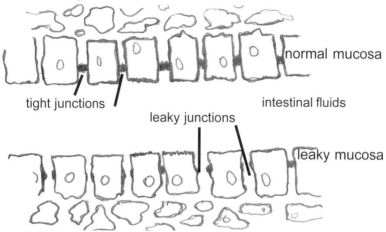

... whilst the bottom row of intestinal cells are leaky. It seems that the chemical "zonulin" determines this leakiness.

The zonulin story

Recently, more information has been discovered about the way the body normally controls the specialized seams between cells (called, "tight-junctions"). Normally, the spaces between gut cells are tightly closed. In some conditions these junctions are too loose, or "leaky". These leaky junctions have been shown to occur in disorders such as diabetes, coeliac disease, and some brain illnesses (Fasano, 2000).

The amount of "between-cell leakiness" is due to a substance called *zonulin*. Both brain tissues and gut tissues contain a cell-surface protein that zonulin binds to. When zonulin binds to these cell receptors, the cells respond by opening their tight junctions. Zonulin is therefore a "key" that opens a gateway, or door, between cells.

Zonulin makes cell junctions more leaky

Complicating matters, there are several versions of zonulin. The zonulin that is made in the intestines differs by a few amino acids from the zonulin that is produced in the brain and in other tissues. These minor alterations in the structure of zonulin are designed to prevent one tissue type (say the gut) from altering the tight junctions of another tissue (say, the brain). These different versions of zonulin makes good biological sense. Your body may need to make your intestine more leaky but, at the same time, keep the blood-brain barrier tight.

In coeliac disease, these gateways between the cells seem to be stuck open. It has been found that gut tissue from people with acute coeliac disease contains much more zonulin than does similar tissue from people who are free of the disease. Gluten appears to stimulate inappropriately high levels of zonulin production. This could explain some of the varied symptoms of coeliac disease. In addition, these leaky tight-junctions in a person with coeliac disease may allow molecules to leak from the intestine into the bloodstream. This process can trigger autoimmune reactions.

Gluten affects the gut

Leaky gut problems

This leaky gut causes a number of problems. First, it permits considerable amounts of these partially digested gluten proteins to get inside the body, through the gut wall. These "foreign" proteins are recognised by your immune system to be invading your body. These proteins are deemed a hazard. So the alarm bells of the immune system ring and an antibody response is triggered.

The purpose of this immune reaction is to rid your body of these foreign proteins. The same mechanism is used to get rid of invading viruses, bugs and germs. Bugs come and assault you, but only *intermittently*. Every now and then they stimulate you to make an immune response, you kill the bug – end of story.

However, there is a huge difference between the gluten and any attacking bugs. By eating gluten every day you are *continuously* challenging your body and so there is a perpetual immune reaction being stimulated.

This can cause both local damage as well as distant problems. In addition, your immune system can get worn down by all of this activity and thus make you more susceptible to other immune attacks. You are literally run-down. You become chronically unwell.

Gluten can make you run-down

This leaky gut condition can occur in a number of ways. Some people have a genetic predisposition to have a leaky gut. Studies show that people with coeliac disease, even properly treated, have a more permeable gut mucosa when compared with normal groups. The data is not yet available for similar measurements on people who are gluten-sensitive without coeliac disease. Perhaps those with naturally leaky guts are the ones who are susceptible to gluten-sensitivity.

Also, when your gut becomes inflamed by infections and other illness, the mucosal permeability also gets increased. This might be from increased zonulin in the gut tissues. This again means that increased amounts of peptides and proteins can now reach the blood stream. I have done studies on children recovering from gastroenteritis (Ford, 1985). Although they are fully recovered within a few days of having a diarrhoea episode, my tests showed that it still took them several days for their gut to recover properly. They had leaky guts for several days or even weeks after the infection had well passed. During such a time of vulnerability, these children might become sensitized to gluten and to other food proteins.

Other conditions that cause gut inflammation are ulcerative colitis and Crohn's disease. In these diseases, the gut is inflamed for a very long time. Again these people are more susceptible to developing gluten-sensitivity. Another effect of a leaky gut is that it lets the gluteomorphines through more easily. So even if there is not an adverse immune response developed against gluten, nonetheless, these morphine-like chemicals can cause stimulation to your brain receptors.

You have now learned a lot about gluten. You also now know that chronic symptoms are very common in so-called "normal" people. The next step is to find out about the problems that gluten can cause.

2. What is gluten-sensitivity?

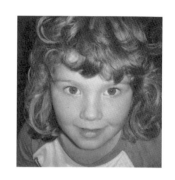

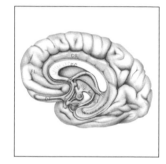

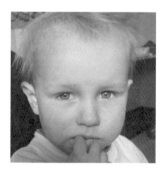

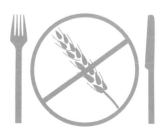

What is gluten-sensitivity?

The term "gluten-sensitive" applies to *any* reaction that is caused by gluten. This includes the many symptoms experienced throughout the gastro-intestinal tract. But it also applies to the host of other non-gastroenterological symptoms. These include brain disorders, skin problems, muscle and joint problems. Gluten-sensitivity occurs ten times more frequently than coeliac disease.

Gluten-sensitivity should be seen as an umbrella term. It includes a wide variety of reactions to gluten. The best recognised manifestation is "coeliac disease" which is an auto-immune condition that destroys the lining of the small intestine. This in turn interferes with nutrient digestion and absorption.

Identify your symptoms

If you have *any* chronic health problems that just won't go away, then you might be gluten-sensitive. The symptoms and health problems of being gluten-sensitive are very wide-ranging. They are listed on the next page. If you can answer "yes" to any of these symptoms, then you might have it.

There is a three-step process to find out if you are affected.
1.   Check out your symptoms.
2.   Get your blood tests.
3.   Interpret your results.
Because there is no single recognisable illness caused by gluten, this entity has been hard to define. This is why these gluten-sensitive problems have been overlooked for so long. However, with the blood tests now available, it has become much easier to diagnose. The world seems to be full of people who are suffering from chronic ill health because of gluten. This book will demonstrate that most of these symptoms can be caused through nerve and brain damage.

Gluten-sensitive problems

Do you or your family have any of these problems?

- ☐ tired and exhausted
- ☐ uncomfortable tummy
- ☐ bloating and gas troubles
- ☐ gastric reflux or heartburn
- ☐ diarrhoea or constipation

- ☐ unhappy with your weight
- ☐ not growing well
- ☐ eating problems
- ☐ lack energy, weakness
- ☐ run-down

- ☐ runny nose and sinus problems
- ☐ chronic iron deficiency
- ☐ osteoporosis or growing pains
- ☐ dermatitis, eczema, itchy or bad skin
- ☐ infertility

- ☐ headaches or migraine
- ☐ feel depressed or moody or grumpy
- ☐ find it hard to think clearly
- ☐ poor sleep

- ☐ hyperactive or cranky
- ☐ Attention Deficit Hyperactivity Disorder (ADHD)
- ☐ autism
- ☐ mental health problems

If you can answer "yes" to any of these problems,
then you or your children could be gluten-sensitive.

The ten target organs

The diagram puts these symptoms in context. I have grouped them into ten "target" organs in your body that can be adversely affected by gluten. Each target organ is indicated by a diamond box. As you can see, the small bowel is only one of these target organs. In this scheme, coeliac disease is considered to be part of the gluten-sensitive spectrum. These ten target organs are:

Gut related symptoms

1. Mouth	– ulcers, runny nose, sore throat.	
2. Oesophagus	– gastro-oesophageal reflux, heart burn, swallowing difficulties.	
3. Stomach	– indigestion, slow emptying, gastritis.	
4. Small bowel	– coeliac disease (enteropathy), malabsorption, diarrhoea.	
5. Colon	– diarrhoea and constipation, bloating, low immune function.	
6. Rectum	– constipation, soiling (encopresis).	

Other symptoms

7. Brain	– disturbed behaviour, migraine, grumpy, tired, headache, depression, mood disorders, ataxia, autism, epilepsy, Attention Deficit Hyperactivity Disorder (ADHD).
8. Skin	– Dermatitis Herpetiformis, eczema.
9. Immune	– run-down, low immunity, recurrent infections.
10. Growth	– poor height and weight (short and/or thin).

Nutritional consequences

In addition to damage to these target organs, there are the nutritional consequences of a poorly functioning gut. These problems include:

Bones and joints	– osteoporosis, bone and joint pain.
Nutritional deficiency	– anaemia, osteoporosis, low levels of vitamins and minerals.
Infertility	

Ten gluten-sensitive target organs

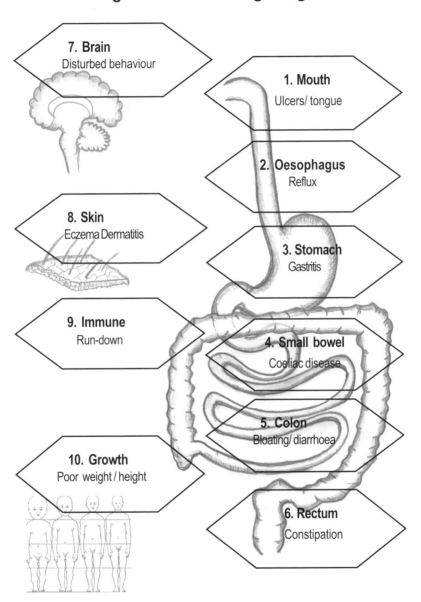

7. **Brain**
Disturbed behaviour

1. **Mouth**
Ulcers/ tongue

2. **Oesophagus**
Reflux

8. **Skin**
Eczema Dermatitis

3. **Stomach**
Gastritis

9. **Immune**
Run-down

4. **Small bowel**
Coeliac disease

5. **Colon**
Bloating/ diarrhoea

10. **Growth**
Poor weight / height

6. **Rectum**
Constipation

43

You cannot tell unless you test!

If you have symptoms that suggest that you might be gluten-sensitive, then you must get your blood tested. You cannot know if your symptoms are caused by gluten until you test for it, especially with the IgG-gliadin test. Do not go gluten-free until you get your blood tests! These are the specific tests that you need:

☐   **IgG-gliadin**   (also called IgG anti-gliadin antibody)
       This test is essential - ask if your lab will do this test.
☐   **IgA-gliadin**   (also called IgA anti-gliadin antibody)
☐   **tTG antibody**   (also called IgA tissue transglutaminase)
       or Endomesial Antibodies (EMA)
☐   **Total IgA antibody levels**
       (looking for deficiency in your IgA antibody production)
☐   **Ferritin**   (this is a measure of your iron stores)
☐   **Hb**   (Haemoglobin to check for anaemia)
☐   **CRP**   (C Reactive-Protein to look for inflammation)

Get the correct interpretation

The next step is to get an accurate interpretation of the meaning of your blood tests. Currently, these tests are often misinterpreted. In particular, the IgG-gliadin levels are often dismissed as being meaningless. However, I believe that this is a crucial measurement and it should be taken very seriously. If you need help with the interpretation of your blood tests, then follow these steps:

1. Get your blood tests and get a copy of these results.
2. Go to the webpage **www.doctorgluten.com**
3. Then, at **Blood Test Results** enter your test results
       (http://www.doctorgluten.com/bloodresults.htm)
4. You will be sent an interpretation of your blood test results with suggestions of what action you should take.

You might have coeliac disease

If you have a high tTG antibody test, this indicates that you probably have significant bowel damage (coeliac disease, also known as gluten sensitive enteropathy). You should have a confirmatory small bowel biopsy. You should seek a gastroenterology opinion. Some laboratories prefer to measure the EMA (Endomesial antibody) level which gives similar information to the tTG results.

Coeliac disease history

Coeliac disease was the first condition recognised as being caused by gluten. It is also called gluten-sensitive enteropathy or even Celiac Sprue. Coeliac disease has a history of over 100 years. The entity of "coeliac disease" was first described by Samuel Gee in 1888. He called it "the Coeliac affection".

Gee had recognised a group of people, particularly children between one and five years old, who had smelly pale bowel motions, who did not look at all well, who had a pot belly, who were fatigued and who did not grow well. He did not know what caused this disease. But he did recognise this as a clinical pattern of what is called "malabsorption". These people had a severe nutritional deficiency and did not live very long.

Coeliac disease is a gut disease

Thus, coeliac disease had been defined as a malabsorption condition. Therefore, coeliac disease is predominantly seen as a gastro-intestinal disease. It is identified when there is damage to the small intestinal mucosa (internal gut skin) from the toxic effects of gluten in the diet. This gut damage is called "villus atrophy".

In 1950, Willem Dicke recognised that this "affection" was a disease caused by the toxic effects of eating gluten. He observed that when these patients were taken off wheat, they quickly recovered. This was a breakthrough, and the pace of understanding quickened.

A few years later, in 1957, Dr Margo Shiner, a Paediatric Gastroenterologist, was the first person to obtain a piece of tissue from the small intestine from a child who had been diagnosed clinically as having coeliac disease. Under the microscope, she found that the skin (mucosa) of the intestine was very abnormal – this appearance was called "villus atrophy". Without such gut damage, coeliac disease is not officially recognised. This gut damage is usually totally reversible with a gluten-free diet.

This tissue damage has subsequently shown to be strongly associated with positive blood tests of Endomysial antibodies (EMA) and tissue transglutaminase antibodies (tTG). It has recently been discovered that coeliac disease is also strongly associated with the HLA types DQ2 and DQ8 (a gene test for coeliac disease).

For nearly a hundred years there has been a narrow focus on coeliac disease as being a gut disease. Thus, the centre of attention of all investigations has been on the presence or absence of bowel damage. Consequently, the adverse reactions to gluten have generally been considered as exclusively gut-related.

This long legacy of focusing on the gut has created a huge barrier for established medical practitioners. They now have great difficulty in widening their view to recognise the many other symptoms that gluten-sensitivity causes.

The great masquerader

Coeliac disease has been called the great masquerader. This is because people with established coeliac disease can have extremely varied symptoms and other associated diseases. The manifestations of coeliac disease extend far beyond the small-bowel tissue.

The medical literature is full of descriptions of disorders that have been shown to be related to the presence of coeliac disease. The conundrum is that these other disorders may not provide any apparent clinical clue that there is underlying coeliac disease. A list of these related conditions is as follows. I have put the neurological conditions at the top as this is the eventual focus of this book.

Brains and nerves

> Peripheral neuropathy and myopathy
> Epilepsy, convulsions
> Ataxia
> Myelopathy
> Psychiatric disturbances
> Depression and mood disorders

Mouth and gut

> Recurrent aphthous mouth ulcers
> Defects in tooth enamel
> Pharyngeal and oesophageal carcinoma
> Reflux oesophagitis
> Lymphocytic gastritis
> Liver disease
> Irritable bowel syndrome
> Ulcerative jejunitis
> Adenocarcinoma of small bowel

Hormones

Type 1 diabetes
Infertility in men and women
Recurrent abortion
Thyroid disorders
Adrenal disorders (Addison's disease)

Blood and immune

Anaemia (iron, folate and vitamin B12 deficiency)
Coagulation disorders from vitamin K deficiency
IgA deficiency
Hyposplenism
T-cell lymphoma
Cardiomyopathy

Bones and joints

Osteopenia
Arthralgia/arthritis
Osteoporosis
Growing pains

Skin and hair

Dermatitis herpetiformis
Eczema
Psoriasis
Brown pigmentation of face and cheek mucosa
Alopecia areata (hair loss)

Genetic

Trisomy 21 (Down's syndrome)

I emphasize, that this list of conditions has been associated with the occurrence of the histological damage in the small bowel that is the hallmark of coeliac disease.

Gluten-sensitivity can cause all of this

But, I go on to argue that these conditions are also associated with the gluten-sensitivity in the absence of gut damage.

Marsh's "modern" definition of gluten-sensitivity

Marsh was the person who, early on, clearly described the histological criteria for making the diagnosis of coeliac disease. The "Marsh" criteria has become the official way of recording the degree of bowel damage caused by gluten. He has subsequently recognised the much wider spectrum of disease that is precipitated by gluten.

In his updated definition (Marsh, 1995) he said, "Gluten-sensitivity is a state of heightened immunological responsiveness to ingested gluten in genetically susceptible individuals. Such responsiveness may find expression in organs other than the gut".

How does the gut damage happen?

Gliadin, one of the principal wheat proteins, seems to be the culprit. Wheat, rye, and barley (and to a minor extent, oats) have progressively lesser amounts of gliadin. It is gliadin that has a toxic amino-acid sequence. Specifically, alpha-gliadin.

When gliadin gets through the leaky gut, it then reacts with the immune system, whose job is to protect you from foreign invaders. The gluten proteins are "presented" to the T-cells which then get switched on or sensitized. This immune reaction, in conjunction with HLA-DQ2 or HLA-DQ8 antigen (why this is so remains a mystery), leads to the production of a collection of chemicals which cause tissue damage. These chemicals are called "cytokines".

The cytokines, as well as causing tissue damage within the mucosa, also start to activate even more immune cells. Next, the antibody producing cells (called "plasma cells") get stimulated to produce antibodies to at least three proteins: to gliadin; to tissue transglutaminase (a tissue enzyme in damaged cells); and to endomysium (a tissue protein). These antibodies can be measured in your blood to see if you are being damaged by gluten.

An explanation about the blood tests

The coeliac and gluten blood test markers have been progressively developed over the last twenty years. This has radically changed the understanding of gluten-sensitivity.

There are two different groups of antibodies

These blood tests can be divided into two groups. They measure quite different phenomena:
o   Gluten (food) antibodies.
o   Tissue (gut damage) antibodies.

Gluten antibodies

The anti-gliadin antibodies (sometimes abbreviated as AGA, or more simply known as "gliadin" antibodies) are antibodies which are directed against gluten or gliadin *in the diet*. Gliadin is a specific protein that is part of gluten. There are two types of these antibodies: IgG-gliadin and IgA-gliadin. These antibodies are made by your immune system against the gluten from wheat, rye and barley.

These blood tests are very sensitive. They detect the immune reaction to gluten. But they are poor predictors of people who have coeliac disease.

Gluten antibodies are diet related

However, these tests are nearly always strongly positive in people with untreated coeliac disease (who are not on a gluten-free diet). On a strict diet, these antibody levels will begin to fall within a few months.

IgA-gliadin antibody: The IgA-gliadin antibody is a useful marker of gluten reactions. However, it does not become positive in everyone who has coeliac disease. If it is elevated, then you are very likely to have symptomatic gluten-sensitivity. This test can be also used for monitoring compliance when on a gluten-free diet. If it stays high, then you are likely to still be consuming significant amounts of gluten.

IgG-gliadin antibody: If there is a lone elevation of IgG-Gliadin, then this usually indicates the development of a gluten-sensitivity. With ongoing eating of gluten, established full-blown coeliac disease could develop over time (years or even decades) in genetically susceptible people. In my experience, the great majority of people who have raised IgG-gliadin antibody tests are gluten-sensitive but do not have coeliac disease.

Currently, laboratories are abandoning this test because it is not specific enough to diagnose coeliac disease. However, it does identify gluten-sensitivity reactions which are ten times more common that coeliac disease.

IgG-gliadin antibody test is a very useful blood test

Tissue antibodies

The Endomysial antibody (abbreviated as EMA) and tissue-transglutaminase antibody (abbreviated as tTG) are directed against the damaged *tissue* of the bowel.

Tissue antibodies are a response to mucosal damage

In coeliac disease, there is an overreaction of the immune system. A harmful immune reaction occurs at the intestinal lining – the mucosa. This involves inflammatory cells, cytokines, and the production of antibodies. This abnormal immune response is triggered by the presence of gliadin.

The tissue damage is the result from ongoing attack by the immune system. It erroneously invades parts of the delicate supporting structures surrounding the muscle fibres in the gut tissue. This structure is called the endomysium. The inflammation in the endomysial tissue results in the production of the anti-endomysial antibodies. This is what the blood test identifies and is the reason why people with coeliac disease (who have damaged small bowel tissue) have antibodies to a muscle tissue (endomysium).

EMA (Endomysial antibody): The endomysium is the delicate tissue that surrounds and supports the muscle fibres. The endomysial antibody (EMA) is an IgA-based antibody. It is an auto-antibody. That means it is an abnormal antibody directed against your own tissues. Until recently, the EMA had been found to be the most specific blood test for screening populations for coeliac disease (damaged bowel). For example, if you want to look at all the people in your town and find out those who have coeliac disease, then the most cost effective way of doing it is by just measuring everybody's EMA levels.

This test generally becomes negative following 12–18 months on a gluten-free diet.

However, there are a number of problems with the EMA test. It is an immuno-histo-chemical assay. It uses either monkey oesophagus or human umbilical cord. The blood sample and chemicals are put onto this tissue and observed under a microscope. Thus the test is prone to technical error, inconsistent results and is time-consuming. Also, in children under two years old this test cannot be relied upon to give an accurate indication of tissue damage.

tTG (tissue Transglutaminase) antibody: There is a special enzyme that is present in muscle tissue – this enzyme is called tissue transglutaminase. It seems that this enzyme can readily combine with gliadin. Somehow, this combination makes tTG more easily recognised by the body's immune system. This was discovered in 1997.

---

tTG antibody accurately indicates tissue damage

Technical note: tTG has been shown to be the antigen that is recognised by endomysial antibodies in people with coeliac disease. Currently, a high level of tTG (tissue transglutaminase) antibody (which is also an IgA based antibody) in the blood is the most accurate blood test to make the diagnosis of coeliac disease in an individual.

If you have got a positive tTG antibody test, then there is about a 95% chance (but still not a 100%) that you will have an abnormal biopsy, with the telltale signs of coeliac disease. IgA antibodies to tTG become negative 9–24 months after commencement of a gluten-free diet.

The measurement of tTG is not without problems. Antigens used in the various test kits vary in their source and also arbitrary units are used to denote the positive value. So these factors contribute to the variations in sensitivity, specificity and predictive values that are reported. tTG can also be positive in other chronic inflammatory conditions. High levels have been reported in association with chronic liver disease and inflammatory bowel disease.

Also, tTG cannot be relied upon to always be present in early coeliac disease in young children, particularly under two years.

Finally, all tests that measure IgA antibodies are of no value in a person who is deficient at producing IgA which is found in about 10% of coeliacs. Therefore, it is important to measure total IgA levels as well as the specific antibodies for an accurate interpretation.

HLA typing

HLA is the abbreviation for the "Histocompatibility Leukocyte Antigen". It is used primarily as a test in tissue typing. It is like an expanded blood-type test. In blood-typing, the main groups are ABO and Rh (positive or negative). However, the HLA typing system is used for other tissues. It is detailed and complex. Of interest, many HLA tissue types have been associated with a great many specific diseases.

It has now been discovered that most patients with biopsy-proven coeliac disease have the HLA class II haplotype: HLA-B8, DR3 (more commonly known as DQ2 and DQ8). Indeed, coeliac disease is rare in people who do not have this tissue type. The "wrong" genes are only found in about 3–5% of coeliacs.

In the general population, about 20% carry this same HLA set. Therefore, other mechanisms must be involved with the development of coeliac disease. Not all HLA DQ2 or DQ8 people will get coeliac disease. There are likely to be additional but as yet unidentified genes involved.

HLA typing has a very useful contribution to make. It is used as another marker of coeliac status. But on its own it cannot be used as a diagnostic test. It is valuable in making a decision on who should have a small bowel biopsy.

What if my blood tests are negative?

From this discussion, it is clear that the blood tests are extremely useful. These antibody blood tests can tell you if you are reacting to gluten and if you have bowel damage.

However, these blood tests are not perfect! In particular, there are a number of children who have all of the clinical symptoms and signs of coeliac disease but they have negative blood tests. These children need to have a small bowel biopsy. The blood tests cannot be totally relied upon.

Blood tests are not infallible

Also, the gluten blood tests are only testing for gliadin antibody reactions. There may be other wheat proteins yet to be recognised that are causing harm but are not yet being tested for.

I have many patients who have normal blood tests and a normal bowel biopsy, but when they have gone on a gluten-free diet they have recovered.

Another problem is the small bowel biopsy. This test is also not a perfect or reliable test. Damage can be patchy and not seen. And when done at a young age, the gluten damage might not be severe enough to see under the microscope. The diagnosis and management of both coeliac disease and gluten-sensitive people is not straight forward. Sometimes, after testing, it is worthwhile going on a gluten-free diet for a trial period. You have nothing to lose – you may gain a great deal.

Small bowel biopsy

The purpose of the small bowel biopsy is to confirm, or diagnose, coeliac disease. It is very important to make an accurate diagnosis for both coeliac disease and gluten-sensitivity. However, a key message of this book is that it is very common to be gluten-sensitive *without* having any bowel abnormalities.

Bowel biopsies can be unreliable

The small bowel biopsy is a simple test to see how much damage there is in the gut. It can help answer the question: "Is it, or is it not, coeliac disease?" However, it cannot either diagnose or refute the diagnosis of gluten-sensitivity. Also, it cannot dismiss the diagnosis of coeliac disease.

A small bowel biopsy is performed using an endoscope. A flexible tube (about as thick as your little finger) is gently put into your mouth and slowly fed into your stomach and eventually to the small bowel. This tube carries a miniature camera and a few instruments. A tiny piece of skin is taken from the upper bowel (this is the "biopsy"), and then the endoscope is removed. The procedure is done under sedation. It only takes about twenty minutes. It is a very safe procedure in healthy people.

At the same time, tissue biopsies can also be taken from the oesophagus (looking for oesophagitis) and from the stomach (looking for gastritis). The damaged bowel in coeliac disease is called *villus atrophy*. With severely damaged gut tissue, your gut is not able to absorb your food nutrients. You are certain to experience nutritional deficiencies.

The disaccharidase test: Information about the function of the small bowel can also be obtained by small bowel biopsy. The disaccharidase tests measure the enzymes that digest sugars in the small intestine. This gives the activity of the lactase, sucrase, and maltase enzymes.

Is there an epidemic?

The extensive data that is now available shows that at least 10% of the population is sensitized to gluten. Some of this evidence comes from population studies measuring IgG-gliadin antibody levels. There is now a large body of evidence from clinical studies that identify gluten-sensitivity as being common.

Population studies on *coeliac disease* (or gluten sensitive enteropathy) have found it to occur in about one in a hundred people.

One in ten are affected by gluten

From my own clinical data, an estimate can be made on the incidence of gluten-sensitivity. I make a diagnosis of gluten-sensitivity ten times more frequently than coeliac disease. The implication of this is that one person in ten is gluten-sensitive. This makes gluten-sensitivity a gigantic health problem. The numbers of people suffering from gluten-sensitivity is in epidemic proportions.

I think that the main reason for the jump in recognition of this problem has been the availability of the blood tests. It can now easily be recognised and diagnosed. I think that this problem of gluten-sensitivity has been with us for a very long time, but only now has it been recognised. However, to understand where we are today requires a trip back to the past.

Free Bonus Chapter

Since the first printing of this book, I have been asked to give a much more detailed explanations of the blood tests and endoscopy results. I am frequently asked about how early coeliac disease can be diagnosed. Also, is gluten-sensitivity permanent? What about the genetic test for coeliac disease and how can the results be used?

To read this bonus chapter, and other bonus material, please go to: http://www.doctorgluten.com/bonus.htm

3. Gluten grains

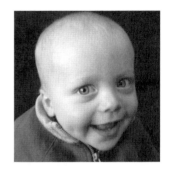

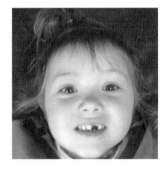

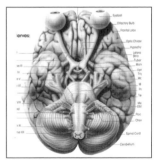

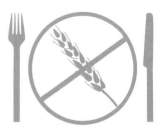

The age of gluten grains

As time has gone by, our diets have slowly become full of it. Full of gluten. This is how it happened.

Hunter Gatherers

A very long time ago, hundreds of thousands of years ago, primitive man was known as a hunter gatherer. This meant that man ate the food that was available on that day, and in that season. Meat was hunted. Fruits, nuts and vegetables were gathered. There was no farming. There was no agriculture. There was no substantial storage. Man was nomadic, living a hand-to-mouth existence.

In these times, their diet was almost devoid of gluten. Small amounts of gluten might have been derived from the gathering of grass seeds. This must have been a tough life. Longevity was not a problem! Life-spans were measured in terms of 15–25 years. Accidents were rife and you could easily be hunted down by a hungry carnivore.

The origins of grains

The dawn of the agriculture mentality appeared about 10,000 years ago. There were wild grasses growing which produced small seeds of grain. There is evidence that these grains were harvested, stored and eaten. The next step in this slow evolution was to keep some of these seeds back for the next season, and then deliberately plant them to harvest the subsequent year.

This development of agriculture could only happen when man had become less nomadic and had began to settle in organised villages. He had to be able to tend and protect his crop. He needed the certainty of staying in one place for many years.

The advantage of growing and harvesting grain was that their food source could at last become more reliable. At last, food was readily available. Also, large quantities could be grown, and this grain was relatively easy to store. This was the beginning of gluten being introduced as a substantial protein in the diet of early man. It was the beginning of the gluten saga.

Grains gave a reliable source of food

Grasses and grains

The very act of picking wild grains and then harvesting them led to progressive changes in these grains. Initially, these grass grains were selected for those that stayed attached to the stalks whilst they were ripening. This meant that collection of the grain seed was more efficient, rather than gathering the fallen seed from the ground. As grains were grown, and then transported from the central African plains to more northern parts of the globe, different characteristics were slowly bred into the grain. The gluten content steadily rose.

It turns out that gluten is an important protein in the wheat seed. It helped the wheat plant grow successfully in the northern cooler regions. This gluten protein has a role in the successful storage and subsequent germination of the wheat seed. Paradoxically, the advantage that gluten conferred for the productive growing of wheat (of being resistant to breakdown), bestowed a great disadvantage to the very people who unceasingly developed it.

Unfortunately, we humans do not have the appropriate digestive enzymes to adequately digest gluten in our gut. So gluten began to undermine the health of susceptible people in the population.

Bread and fast-foods

Over the last 5,000 years, the amount of gluten in the western diet has steadily increased. Bread has become the staple diet. However, in the last 50 years this whole process has accelerated.

Gluten has a number of properties that has made its wide scale use inevitable. Gluten is a protein that gives a pleasing texture and flavour to bread. Gluten is a stringy elastic protein that helps bind wheat starch in a way that traps air. This allows the bread to be baked more spongy, light and chewy. This is a property that is prized by bakers. It allows the bread to have more volume.

Because gluten-rich grains are valued by the bread industry, there has been pressure on the agriculture sector to develop and harvest grains that have an even higher gluten content. This gives better visco-elastic properties. With a sophisticated understanding of food technology and breeding programs, gluten-rich grains are now the norm.

We eat vast amounts of gluten

A further step in this chain of events has been the development of fast-food outlets. These meals on buns, on breads and on pizza bases are all made from gluten-rich flour. This has greatly increased the overall gluten intake of modern man. Added to this, there is rampant overeating and huge serving sizes (super-sizing) which yet again increases the amount of gluten being consumed. Because wheat-based gluten foods are relatively cheap, this has also limited the range of foods that are readily available. Nowadays, there is a tendency for people to eat only a narrow range of foods. Subsequently, as a nation we are eating more gluten-foods and less fruits and vegetables.

The food pyramid

The final victory for gluten has been the concept of the food pyramid. Over the last few decades, the recommended pattern of eating has been described as a food pyramid. The bottom of the pyramid comprises grains and breads. The recommendation is for people to eat the highest proportion of their food from gluten-grains! This official sanction of these grains has made them appear to be harmless. It is only recently that the harm from gluten has become apparent.

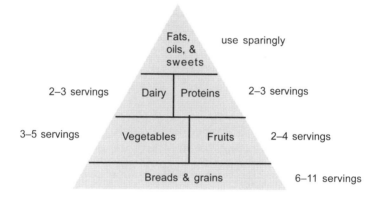

This is the "pyramid" advice that is currently in vogue:
"Breads, grains, cereals and pastas provide complex carbohydrates, which are an important source of energy. You need 6 to 11 servings of these foods in a day. One serving of this group can be: 1 slice of bread; or 1/2 cup of rice; or ½ cup cooked cereal or pasta; or 1 cup of ready-to-eat cereal; or 1 flat bread."

This is often modified to sound more healthy:
"Try to eat whole-grain breads, cereal and pasta for most of your servings from this group. Whole-grain foods (which are made with whole wheat flour) are less processed and retain more valuable vitamins, minerals and fibre than foods made with white flour."

So, at present, the foundation of the official recommended diet is grain-based. And most of the grains are gluten-rich grains. The tragedy is that one in ten people are now suffering from the adverse effects of gluten, but they are unaware of this.

Acidophilus activity

The last straw is the depletion of healthy bacteria in your gut. These good bacteria, called lactobacillus acidophilus and the bifido-bacteria species, are very important passengers living in your large bowel. These bugs help you have a healthy colon and help you with your immune function. They also play a part in the control of the leakiness of your gut mucosa. These bacteria are being depleted because of the antiseptics and antibiotics that are now so common in your environment and your food chain.

The shocking truth

All of these factors have contributed to this "epidemic" of gluten-sensitivity. It has been slowly mounting. It has only recently been discovered because of the antibody blood tests that are now available.

The implications for health and sickness prevention are enormous. The health burden of gluten-sensitivity could be so easily lifted as soon as the reluctant health professional get behind this concept. The cost/benefit issues for health are obvious. However, there is likely to be a big opposition camp in the grain and wheat processing industries.

The shocking truth behind gluten is that its toxic effect goes almost unrecognised. People are told to just accept and put up with their symptoms. The horror is that it can attack your brain, your nerves and your mind. We are now going to look at how these gluten-grains can cause this damage to your brain.

4. Your tummy brain

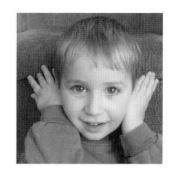

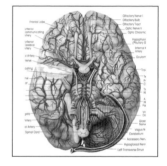

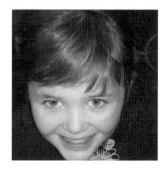

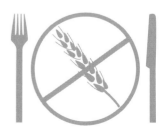

Your tummy brain

Eating should be both pleasurable and comfortable for you. If not, then there is something wrong with you. It is my belief that gluten can strike you down by interfering with your nervous system. How have you been struck by it?

Your gut is full of nerves. Your "tummy brain" refers to the huge networks of nerves cells and nerve fibres that lace through your gastro-intestinal tract (your gut). Your brain is inextricably linked to your gut. Your thoughts and emotions will affect your gut. And the other way round, your gut can affect your brain.

What is your gut doing?

If your gut is functioning normally, then you should be mostly unaware of it. Under normal circumstances you cannot tell that your gut is doing anything! Under normal circumstances, your body tells you that you need to eat – by giving you a sensation of hunger. When you respond by eating something, you are aware of the taste. You also experience the chewing and the swallowing. Otherwise, you should be mostly unaware of your digestive process.

Being normal is to be unaware of your gut

At the end of all of this digestion, your gut gives you the final signal – that is the signal to empty your bowel and defecate. You should have no sensation of your gut's activities in between swallowing and evacuating. In fact, in between the chewing and the down-loading, your gut has been very busy! For those who want to know more about the basic physiology of digestion, the next few pages tell you what is happening.

Oesophagus

Your **oesophagus** (also know as your gullet) is the tube that goes from your mouth to your stomach. It pushes your food down by a rhythmical contraction of its muscles. This creates a wave of energy – similar to a snake moving a swallowed egg down its insides. A sort of Mexican-wave of muscle activity. This should be a one-way journey unless you have a vomiting attack.

Reflux is a gluten symptom

But many people experience episodes of "reflux", which is when some of the acid contents from the stomach gets pushed back up into the oesophagus. This can cause a sensation of burning or pain called "heart burn". Acid burps, indigestion and regurgitation are other ways to describe this. Reflux happens when the oesophagus muscles do not work in unison together. The food is supposed to be kept in the stomach by a tight ring of muscle (the lower oesophageal sphincter) at the far end of the oesophagus. Gluten can interfere with these complex muscle mechanisms, disturbing the smooth functioning of swallowing.

Stomach

When your food reaches your **stomach**, it stimulates strong acid to be produced. Primarily, this acid is made to kill any harmful bugs (bacteria) that may be in your food. This is to prevent them from invading you: it is a very effective barrier to bugs. This acid is made in the "parietal cells" in the stomach lining. Like so many activities of the gut, these parietal cells are stimulated by both nerves and chemicals. The chemical "histamine" promotes the acid secretion, and the hormone "gastrin" regulates the amount of acid that is produced.

Stomach nerves: On top of this chemical and hormone stimulus, the nerve networks also influence acid production. If you just think about food (imagine a juicy lemon) your saliva glands begin to make your mouth water and your stomach will begin to produce acid. Just by thinking about food will start your digestive system to get ready for the food to be swallowed.

Chemical and nerve networks control your gut

These nerves also start the stomach to churn and the intestines to begin their squirming. The stress hormones (adrenaline and cortisone) can also activate all of these systems. So all of these symptoms can be triggered by stress as well. This can explain the butterflies in your stomach. As stress levels increase, the heightened gut activity can lead to nausea, cramps, bloating and diarrhoea.

Intrinsic factor: Your stomach also produces the all important "intrinsic factor". This is essential for life because it binds with the vitamin B12 that you get with your food. This "complex" (that is the intrinsic factor linked to B12) eventually gets absorbed in the last part of your small bowel (the ileum). If your stomach cannot produce intrinsic factor, then you are completely unable to absorb any B12. This will cause the condition called pernicious anaemia. The B12 vitamin is part of the red blood cell production chain. You get weak, sick and tired.

Stomach enzymes: Your stomach is a storage container for your swallowed food, which slowly gets ground up and mixed with more enzymes. These peptic enzymes continue the food digestion process. The chewed food gets progressively broken down to smaller and smaller fragments.

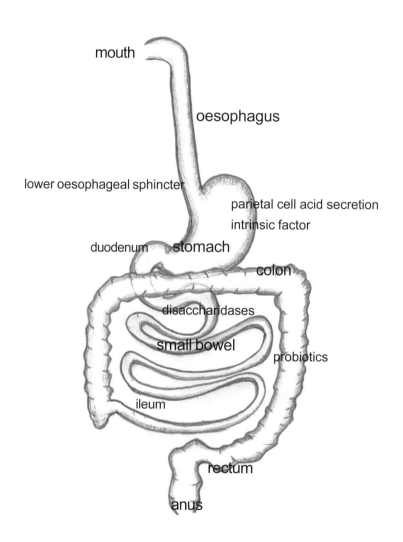

This pulverized digestive mush is then oozed out of your stomach to continue its digestion in the small bowel. Fatty meals slow up this emptying.

Gluten upsets your stomach

Gluten can upset this delicate process, causing your stomach to malfunction. The end result can be reflux, abdominal pain, nausea and indigestion.

Small bowel

The stomach slowly empties this mashed up food, bit by bit, into your small intestine. It is here that the goodness (the nutrients) of your food is absorbed. The small bowel (also called the small intestine) is the main digestive part of your gut. It is a system of very complicated processes that work in harmony together. This is coordinated by the nerve networks and hormone messaging.

Additional enzymes are poured into the small bowel from the gall bladder (producing bile, to digest fats) and from the pancreas (producing specialized enzymes, to digest fats, starch and proteins). The sugar enzymes (called disaccharidases) are manufactured on the surface layer of the small bowel mucosa.

Your small bowel absorbs the food nutrients

All of this activity is focused on the rapid break down of the food into its component parts. Only then can these precious nutrients get absorbed to maintain your body's healthy functions.

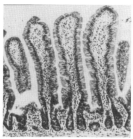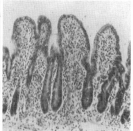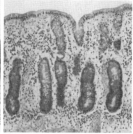

These three pictures are from small bowel biopsies of people being investigated for coeliac disease. The first is an example of a *normal* small bowel biopsy (it shows the long finger-like villi and the crypt structure). The other two show abnormal mucosa with shortened villi and deepened crypts. They show *subtotal villus atrophy* and *total villus atrophy*.

When your small bowel malfunctions, you cannot extract the goodness of your food – this is the cause of "malabsorption". When that happens, much of the food's nutrients will pass right through you. You can lose fats, proteins, sugars, minerals and vitamins. This makes your faeces abnormal. This loss of vital nutrients makes you sick. In coeliac disease, this damage to the small bowel leads to a wide number of nutritional deficiencies.

The fat break

Your body is an extremely efficient machine. It does not want to waste any food nutrients, especially fat. Fat is highly prized by your body, so it is completely digested and absorbed. Your gut control is very sensitive to the amount of fat both in your meals and in your intestines. High fat meals will slow down your stomach emptying. Further on in the small intestine, food will not be moved on into your colon until every bit of fat has been absorbed. This slow-down is called the "ileal brake". It appears that this sensing of unabsorbed fat occurs at the far end of the bowel, a section called the "ileum". Thus, adjusting your fat intake will alter the speed of food processing inside your gut.

Large bowel

The large bowel (also called the colon) is the last section of your gut. It is here you process the waste material – faeces or poos. The proper efficient functioning of your colon is critical for you to feel comfortable. An important function of the colon is the reabsorption of much of the water that is now in your gut. It also lubricates itself with large amounts of slimy mucous.

The colon is teeming with trillions of bacteria (bugs) that process the fibre content of your diet. Some vitamins are actually manufactured by these bacteria. Also, the "Lactobacillus acidophilus" bacteria live here. They are an essential component of a healthy functioning immune system. These good bugs are known as "probiotics".

Gluten can constipate

The progress of these waste materials downward through the colon is yet again regulated by the nerve networks. It is propelled along by a series of big peristaltic contractions of the strong colon muscles.

Rectum

Finally, your bowel motions are stored in your rectum and expelled through the anus. Constipation can easily occur if there are any glitches throughout the system. For instance, if there is a malfunction of the local neural network, or if there is a central nervous system upset higher up in your brain. Then you can get blocked up. Also, there is a very important contribution to regular bowel motions by the composition of your diet. More fibre is usually good.

When the time finally comes to evacuate this waste material, your consciousness is again aroused and you get the message to download. This is yet another signal that is dependent upon an intact and functional neural network. Many people with chronic constipation do not get this signal to push. They do not easily relax their rectal sphincter. Gluten can hijack this process.

Your gut is a very complex system

In summary, your gut is a long tube that sequentially processes your food. Each part is critical. An intact gut mechanism is absolutely essential to keep you alive and well. Everything that you put in your mouth eventually gets processed: it is either absorbed or excreted. The only control that you have on your body, from the point of view of food, is to decide what you put in your mouth. Once you have swallowed it, and it is in your stomach, then your body takes over.

If you are malabsorbing your food, then more fat will pass straight through you. Any fat in the faeces makes it pale and smelly. Also, it will float in the toilet pan. This type of stool is called steatorrhoea, which is a classical symptom of malabsorption.

Your healthy gut function relies upon a complex series of coordinated activities: an appropriate intake of good foods; a healthy brain and nervous system; the proper excretion of digestive enzymes; and intact immune and hormone systems. My theory is that gluten can undermine many links in this process and start a chain-reaction of physiological havoc.

73

What is your brain doing?

In order to research the wonders of the human body, science has progressively compartmentalized the individual organs and functions of the body into smaller and yet smaller categories. This has led to a much better understanding of workings of each of these individual parts. However, this partitioning has resulted in the isolation of research findings within medical specialties.

Your brain controls your gut

It seems to have been overlooked that your brain plays a vital role in each and every organ of your body. Although your symptoms may be experienced in your gut, or your muscles, or your skin, the primary damage could very well be inside your brain.

How does your brain control your gut?

Your brain has a huge number of roles in the digestion process. Mostly we just take this for granted. Most of our internal activities carry on without us having any perception of it. But when it does go wrong, then you are the first person to know about it!

Your brain has about 25 billion neurons, talking across over 100 trillion synapses, along over 100 million metres of nerve axons. This is some neural network. All of this is contained in your skull and spinal cord – just five kilograms of tissue. Amazing!

Astonishingly, your "tummy brain" has equal numbers of nerve cells and nerve fibres. It is a miracle! Your head brain and your tummy brain work together to get the job done. However, they both have some measure of independence.

Consciousness

Conventionally, our brain function has been subdivided into conscious and unconscious activity. In relation to your gut, your brain has these *conscious* activities:

> Choice of foods
> Feeding yourself
> Cerebral activity before eating (thinking about food)
> Smell taste and texture
> Chewing and swallowing
> Emptying the rectum (defecate).

Most of your gut function is unconscious

But there is a big gap in your awareness whilst your food is being processed and digested. This is the part when your brain is carrying out its *unconscious* activities. Hormone production and regulation is an important part of this phase. This unconscious activity includes:

> Peristalsis to constantly move food along
> Oesophagus – movement
> Stomach – acid and enzyme production and movement
> Small bowel – enzymes and movement
> Gall bladder making bile and contractions
> Pancreas enzyme release
> Large bowel movements
> Rectum storage.

Over the page is a diagram of this very complex network of nerves that controls every facet of your gut function. It is part of the autonomic nervous system – your tummy brain.

Autonomic nervous system

The "autonomic nervous system" is the label used to describe the nerves that are connected to your gut, your heart and your glands. This nervous network is shown in the diagram. These special nerves emerge from the spinal cord at each spinal level, between each vertebra. They are shown in the diagram as a lacework of thin black lines going to all of the internal organs. (The white nerves, also emerging from the spinal cord are those that will go to the muscles and the skin).

The autonomic system runs automatically – hence its name! Because this system runs automatically, you cannot control it by your thoughts. It works through the unconscious part of your brain. However, your emotions do have a very big influence on this system. This system converts your emotions into bodily symptoms and feelings. The organs that are under the command autonomic system include:

> Cardiovascular – heart and blood vessels
> Gut – intestines and bowel
> Bladder and uterus
> Glands – pancreas, gall bladder, sweat, saliva.

These organs are all connected by the vast nerve networks of the tummy brain. These are called involuntary systems because of the lack of any deliberate thought-generated activity.

Sympathetic and Parasympathetic

The autonomic system is subdivided into two distinct parts: the "Sympathetic" and "Parasympathetic" divisions. This distinction is important because these two divisions use different neurotransmitters to pass on their messages. These two divisions balance each other – they can be seen as "yin and yang". They have almost opposite effects from each other.

Nerve networks of the tummy brain

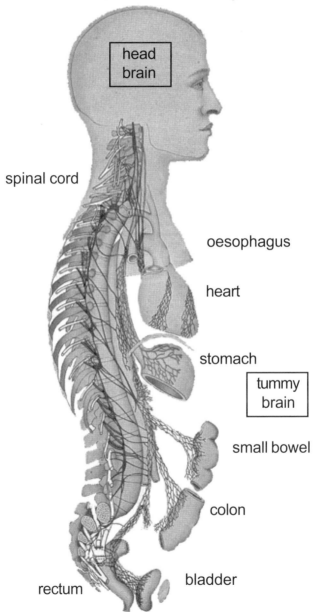

head brain

spinal cord

oesophagus

heart

stomach

tummy brain

small bowel

colon

bladder

rectum

Autonomic symptoms

These opposing activities are listed in the table. The "Sympathetic system" has *stress* activity – driven by the nerve transmitter called norepinephrine (or noradrenaline).

You will be most familiar with the "stress" side of this system. A little bit of stress is exciting and fun. But too much stress puts the body into overload. Looking down the "stress" column you can see that in a highly stressed state you will be flushed, have a fast heart rate and high blood pressure. Your tummy will churn and squirm. You will lose your appetite. You may feel nauseated and get abdominal cramps. Constipation or diarrhoea is common.

In your head you will get feelings of anxiety and fear. Long term this is debilitating and leads to chronic anxiety, depression and poor health. There is also evidence that your immune mechanisms do not work so well in this high stress condition.

On the other hand, the parasympathetic system does the opposite. It balances the sympathetic stress. It should be your default status. The "Parasympathetic system" has a more *relaxing* nature. Its neurotransmitter is acetylcholine. It promotes gastric secretion, bile release into the intestine and promotion of digestive enzymes. However, too much parasympathetic drive does create symptoms. You may get loose bowel motions or even diarrhoea. Your appetite will increase. However, the "stress" side of this system is usually dominant.

The "symptoms" caused by unopposed sympathetic autonomic activity, as you can see, comprise most of the symptoms that have been associated with gluten-sensitivity. This is further circumstantial evidence that the damage caused by gluten is somehow mediated via the autonomic nervous networks.

Symptoms and signs that can be generated through the autonomic nervous system

Organ	Stress Sympathetic symptoms	Relaxing Parasympathetic symptoms
Final nerve ending transmitter	Norepinephrine	Acetylcholine

Cardiovascular – heart and blood vessels

Blushing	Normal	Flushing
Heart rate	Fast	Slow
Blood pressure	High	Normal/ low
	Dizzy	Normal

Gut – intestines and bowel

Appetite	Decreased	Increased
Stomach	Slow emptying	Normal emptying
	Nausea, churning	Normal
	Reflux	Normal
Intestines	Constipation	Diarrhoea
	Bloating	Normal

Glands

Pancreas	Slow	Normal
Sweat glands	Sweaty skin	Dry skin
Saliva	Dry mouth	Saliva produced

Other

Bladder	Empty bladder	Relax bladder
Uterus	Infertility	Fertile

Gut feelings

We all know what gut feelings are. There are two meanings.

First, there are the butterflies in your stomach, the churning of your gut and the feeling of dread in the pit of your tummy. These are emotions that you are feeling in your gut. As the intensity of your emotion increases, your gut will get progressively more distressed. You may eventually feel nausea and even vomit. You may have bloating and distension. You may have diarrhoea.

Your "vagus nerve" is to blame. It is represented by the thick line in the diagram connecting the frontal lobes of your brain to your gut. This vagus nerve is one of the so called "cranial nerves". It is the tenth cranial nerve which has its origins from just under your centre of thought – your frontal lobes. It is able to influence your gut activity in line with your emotions. It works in conjunction with the sympathetic nervous system.

Emotions affect your gut

Second, there are the gut feelings of when you rely on intuition When you have a hunch or when you are inspired. Without thinking something through, you just know what to do. This is your unconscious mind surfacing and giving you complete answers. Sometimes this experience is associated with excitement and good gut feelings. The state of your gut is a mirror of your emotions. In these circumstances, these feelings are channelled through the parasympathetic system. The vagus nerve will also be playing a part in this.

The vagus nerve is a direct link between your brain and your gut.

The vagus nerve – linking brain thought to the gut

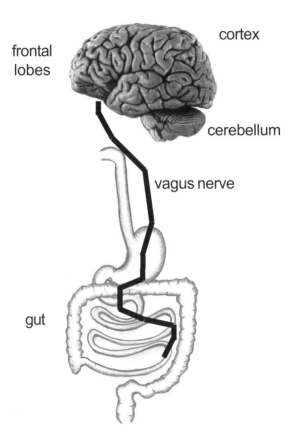

Fight and flight

The fight/flight function of your brain is a survival strategy. It is a deep-seated automatic program that your brain runs to keep you alive when there is an immediate threat to your life. For example, if you are being threatened by a wild animal, you have two choices: to flee; or to stand your ground and fight to the death. Under both of these circumstances you need to act quickly and decisively. You need courage and strength. At this crucial time, adrenaline kicks in. This hormone chemical ramps up all of your systems and gives you heaps of nervous energy. This is the sympathetic nervous system at full throttle. Incredible feats can be achieved under such stress. In the wild, stresses were periodic. In between clashes there was calm.

Constant stress

In our brave new world, we are now likely to be stressed for greater amounts of the time. There are work pressures, family pressures and financial pressures. These can cause ongoing and permanent stress. This keeps the sympathetic nervous system in high gear all of the time. This has a massive detrimental affect on your gut. To be able to function normally it needs to be in the parasympathetic relaxed state.

Worry tummy

This stress and worry is felt in your tummy: gastric reflux, squirming intestines and a bloated gut. Chronic anxiety can lead to vomiting and diarrhoea. Headaches and migraines knock you down.

In my clinical experience, gluten can upset your autonomic nervous system balance. I think that gluten-sensitivity can damage the working of this nerve network. Gluten-sensitivity can present itself through all of these symptoms. Let us look at the details.

5. Gluten strikes your brain

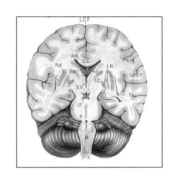

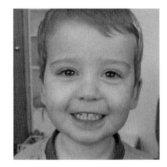

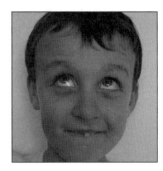

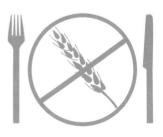

Gluten strikes your brain

My hypothesis is that gluten primarily strikes at the brain. The evidence of how gluten damages the brain comes from a number of directions:

o   Symptoms from the target organs
o   Specific neurological conditions
o   Brain imaging studies
o   Direct microscopic examination of brain cells.

The evidence from "brain symptoms" is overwhelming. There are so many people with "brain symptoms" that are associated with gluten ingestion. This sort of evidence is usually considered to be circumstantial evidence. However, there is a great deal of this type of evidence.

The brain-imaging and brain-cell evidence is found in lesser amounts, but squarely puts the damage in the neural tissues. However, by the time the damage in the brain is so severe that it shows up on special brain x-rays, there is little hope the disease will respond well to a gluten-free diet.

Early diagnosis may prevent later brain damage

I believe that the secret is to recognise the problem early and treat it before any irreversible nerve damage might occur. This evidence will now be presented in detail. In addition, relevant clinical stories are included to put these symptoms into context. I have been convinced that gluten causes major problems with the brain and the nervous networks of the gut.

Symptom evidence

The previous chapter showed the brain has a crucial role in the control of the gut and other organs. So, evidence that gluten-sensitivity is a brain problem should be able to be derived from data from the gluten-sensitive target organs. The brain has thousands of very specific functions which are each housed in specific small, discrete, areas of the brain. For example, the control of your main muscles groups that you can voluntarily move (for instance, moving your right arm) is housed in a specific "motor" segment of your brain cortex. However, the control over your internal organ muscles (for instance, your gut) is housed in your cerebellum.

Gluten-brain connection reports

The first report about neurological disorders that were associated with adult coeliac disease was published in 1966 (Cooke and Thomas-Smith). Most such case reports are usually about people who have had coeliac disease, but then a while later go on to develop some sort of neurological dysfunction. The underlying argument of these reports is that the gut disease is a prerequisite for any subsequent neurological problem.

Brain malfunction with gluten is common

But, thirty years later, a group from the Department of Neurology, Royal Hallamshire Hospital, Sheffield showed that neurological dysfunction can not only precede coeliac disease, but can also be its *only* manifestation (Hadjivassiliou, 1996). Now, a further ten years later, gluten-sensitivity, *without* histological gut damage, is being shown to cause neurological dysfunction. The evidence of gluten-sensitivity as a brain disease is steadily growing.

This is the list of *neurological* conditions that have now been documented to be associated with gluten:

Brain dysfunction

o   Headaches and Migraine
o   Cerebellar ataxia
o   Myoclonic ataxia
o   Chronic neuropathies
o   Autonomic neuropathy
o   Epilepsy
o   Dementia

Mood and Behaviour problems

o   Anger
o   Learning disorders
o   Lethargy, low energy
o   Attention-deficit/hyperactivity disorder (ADHD)
o   Autism
o   Depression
o   Psychiatric disorders
o   Schizophrenia
o   Multiple Sclerosis

Growth and development malfunction

o   Myopathy
o   Poor growth – growth hormone suppression

Gut problems

o   Reflux
o   Constipation
o   Diarrhoea
o   Abdominal pain

The evidence for these disorders will be discussed in detail with relevant illustrated stories. These problems are seen both in coeliac disease and in gluten-sensitivity without intestinal damage.

Neurological findings common

A study has closely investigated the link between coeliac disease and brain malfunction (Zelnik, 2004). Patients with coeliac disease were asked to fill in a questionnaire regarding the presence of neurological disorders or symptoms. Their medical charts were also reviewed.

All those who reported having any neurological manifestations were further studied. They all had an extensive neurological examination. They also had brain imaging studies (brain scans) and an electroencephalogram (EEG), if required. Their neurological information was then compared with that of a control group, which was matched for age and gender.

Half of coeliacs have neurological disorders

They found that their patients who had coeliac disease were very much more likely to have developed neurological disorders (51.4%) in comparison with the control subjects (19.9%).

These neurological disorders included: hypotonia, developmental delay, learning disorders and ADHD (attention deficit hyperactivity disorder), headache, and cerebellar ataxia. Epileptic disorders were only marginally more common.

Next, they were all put on gluten-free diets. But, the therapeutic benefit of a gluten-free diet was only demonstrated in patients with transient infantile hypotonia and migraine headache. They concluded that their study had found that the extent of neurological disorders that occurred in coeliac disease was much broader than had been previously reported. Over a half were affected.

They went on to say that future longitudinal prospective studies were necessary to more fully define the full range of these neurological disorders and their clinical response to a gluten-free diet.

Gluten causes lots of neurologic problems

Poor response to gluten-free diets

A previous in-depth review of the medical literature (Wills, 2000) stated that a number of neurological syndromes had been described in association with coeliac disease.

He said, "that these included disorders of the central nervous system encompassing epilepsy, myoclonus, ataxia, internuclear opthalmoplegia, multifocal leukoencephalopathy and dementia." He went on to say, "most of these associated conditions show a poor response to gluten restriction."

Early diagnosis is the key

However, it has been found that the peripheral neuropathies (of axonal and demyelinating types) may respond to elimination of gluten from the diet.

As I have stated previously, it is not surprising that a gluten-free diet had failed to reverse established neurological damage. Early diagnosis and management must be the key. Once permanent damage has been caused in the brain, it is too late to repair it. Children appear to respond to the benefits of a gluten-free diet more rapidly and more completely than do adults.

Auto-antibody damage

The mechanisms (or causes) of this nerve damage are generally thought to be through autoimmune damage. There is now quite a lot of evidence for this "auto-antibody" damage theory. This is when your own immune system begins to damage your own tissues. A number of nerve and brain antibodies have been detected.

Gluten stimulates the immune system

For example, one study demonstrated "anti-ganglioside" antibodies in 65% of patients with coeliac disease who had also been troubled with some sort of neuropathy. These auto-antibodies have been shown to bind to a number of critical nerve sites that will go on to damage the nerve. These antibodies have been shown to attack the "Schwann cell" surface (this is part of the protective coat of the nerve) and also axons in peripheral nerves (the axon in the main trunk line of the nerve).

In summary, peripheral nerve damage is seen in coeliac disease and various mechanisms have been demonstrated. Gluten-free diets do help many of these patients. It is my belief that gluten-sensitivity (without established coeliac disease) can also manifest all of these symptoms.

Gluten damage

The next piece of information that we need is the actual mechanism by which gluten can inflict so much damage throughout the brain and nervous system. There are a number of candidates for this, of which some or all may play a part As you know, I now think that gluten-sensitivity is mostly a neurological disease. A major contribution to this theory has been the realization that the brain has a central role in the expression of the symptoms that have until now been simply attributed to the local gut toxicity of gluten.

Brain damage can cause gut damage

Traditionally, gluten reactions have been thought to be from gluten directly damaging the gut tissue. However, all of these symptoms can equally be explained through their brain connections and the subsequent disordered feedback mechanisms.

I propose that gluten-sensitivity is both a brain and nervous system disease. But how is the damage caused? There is a gigantic network of nerves that controls every function of your gut. If this network gets damaged, then the gut will malfunction.

Gluten causing inflammation

An inflammatory reaction to gluten in and around the nerve tissues is the mostly likely explanation for the ongoing neuronal malfunction. There is quite a lot of evidence for this.

Gluten can cause nerve cell inflammation

When gluten gets into the body, it stimulates the production of the gluten antibodies by the immune system. The next phase is the formation of "gluten/gluten-antibody" immune complex reactions. This may start off as a non-specific inflammatory reaction, but nerve tissue is very sensitive to surrounding inflammatory activity.

Excitotoxins

The activity of excitotoxins is another factor that could invoke neurological damage. Excitotoxins are biochemical substances (usually amino acids) that can react with special neuronal receptors called "glutamate receptors". This can happen both in the brain and in the spinal cord. This type of reaction is harmful (note that these substances are toxins). It can cause injury or even death to neurons.

These chemicals are called excitotoxins because they are neurotransmitters (such as glutamate or aspartate) which in too higher levels can excite the nerves to death. It is therefore crucial that the levels of these neurotransmitters are regulated properly.

Nerve cells can be excited to death

In a normally functioning nerve, if a high level of these neurotransmitters is generated, then they are re-converted to the more calming neurotransmitter, called GABA. But in the inflamed state, this might not happen.

The way that the nerve death occurs is that the excess of these excitotoxins causes an imbalance in the flow of calcium into the nerve cell. This leads to the activation of an inflammatory cascade, and the subsequent release of even more inflammatory substances. This leads to neural malfunction and eventual nerve cell death.

It is possible that gluten or the "gluten/antibody immune complex" might disturb this delicate balance.

Interfering with neurotransmitters

Secretin is a gut hormone that has a central role in messaging between the nerve cells in the gut. However, secretin is perhaps best known in its role to stimulate the pancreas to release bicarbonate to neutralize the acid which the stomach has produced.

Secretin has been shown to cross the blood/brain barrier which may regulate cells nearby to produce GABA, the calming neurotransmitter. In addition, secretin appears to activate neurons in the amygdala, an area of the brain that integrates social and emotional stimuli. It is possible that gluten may interfere with the secretin receptor or messaging activity.

To date, the effects of gluten on nerve tissue functions have not really been investigated. So at this stage, any "neurotoxic" effect of gluten in speculative. However, there is plenty of objective evidence that brain and nerve damage does occur in association with gluten ingestion. In the following chapters abundant evidence is presented concerning brain damage, which has been directly studied with special x-ray tests of the brain.

Also there is actual brain cell evidence. Some evidence of brain damage has been obtained from an examination of the brain tissue under the microscope. This is called histology or pathology. If there is damage in parts of the brain that control the gut, then it can be inferred that the gut symptoms are directly due to the brain damage rather than gluten acting on the gut.

Next we are going to look at the evidence of gluten as the underlying cause for headaches and migraine.

6. Headaches and migraine

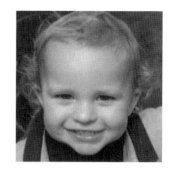

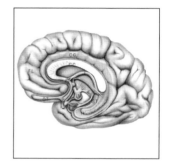

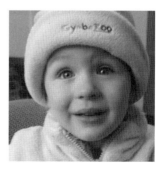

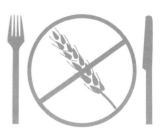

Headaches and migraines

Headaches and migraines have repeatedly been reported to be associated with gluten in the diet. Not surprisingly, researchers have found that removing or cutting back on gluten in the diet can greatly reduced these symptoms.

Medical evidence

One study (Hadjivassiliou, 2001) reported the findings in ten patients with gluten-sensitivity. Their brain tests (MRI-Magnetic Resonance Imaging) had suggested inflammation of their central nervous system. All of these people had experienced significant chronic headaches. Some had also suffered from unsteadiness and poor muscle coordination.

Headache relief off gluten

The great news for them was that after removing gluten from their diets, all of the nine who went gluten-free had full or partial relief (there was only one patient who would not try the diet).

One of these patients tells his story. He was a 50-year-old man who had complained of headaches and nausea along with confusion and agitation. He initially had experienced intermittent severe headaches for four years but then his attacks got even worse, both in frequency and severity. He was delighted that soon after starting a gluten-free diet he became symptom free. His balance improved rapidly and his headaches cleared completely! After going back on gluten, his headaches returned.

Another of these patients was a 45-year-old man. He had suffered from migraine since he was a child. Over time, his attacks had become more and more severe and resisted every treatment. He had blood tests that showed him to be gluten-sensitive. With the introduction of a gluten-free diet, his headaches completely disappeared. There are hundreds of similar cases in which gluten has been shown to be "the trigger factor".

Gluten recognised as the trigger

A different focus of some studies has been to look at the association between headache and coeliac disease. In one study (Gabrielli, 2003), a total of 90 patients affected by migraine (of unknown cause) were enrolled, and compared with 236 blood donors. Four (4.4%) of 90 migraine patients were found to have coeliac disease compared with only 0.4% blood donor controls. This was a highly significant difference – that is a ten times difference. These four people were put on a gluten-free diet for the next six months with impressive results. One of the four patients had no more migraine attacks. The remaining three patients experienced an improvement in frequency, duration, and intensity of their migraine. In summary, of those suffering with migraine, coeliac disease was found in 4.4% of the migraineurs compared with only 0.4% in blood donors.

Migraine people more likely to have coeliac disease

Brain blood flow

This study went on to investigate whether there were any regional cerebral blood-flow abnormalities in migraine patients with coeliac disease. This is because migraine is associated with changes in brain blood-flow. Brain scans were done (a single photon emission CT brain study) on these migraine patients before and after being on a gluten-free diet. Their first brain scan tests showed a regional reduction in blood-flow in all four patients. But this blood-flow reduction was completely reversed at the follow-up brain scan after six month on a gluten-free diet.

Gluten-free diets improved brain blood flow

They concluded that a significant proportion of patients with migraine may have coeliac disease, and that a gluten-free diet may lead to an improvement in the migraine in these patients. A very high prevalence of headache (migraine and/or tension headaches) was also found in coeliac disease patients (46%) when compared with a control group (29%) (Cicarelli, 2003).

Again, looking at coeliac disease, headache was the most common neurological condition in those who had been diagnosed in childhood: 27.9% compared with only 8.1% of a control comparison group. Importantly, about half of these neurological symptoms disappeared when on a gluten-free diet (Zelnik, 2004).

Some of these patients with migraine-like headaches have been shown to have cerebral calcification when studied with head MRI scans. This is probably from long-standing disease. Again I say, the earlier that gluten-sensitivity is diagnosed, the less likely it is going to progress to long-term irreparable damage. Overall, children respond more quickly than adults to a gluten-free diet.

People tell their stories

Here are a few case stories of headaches related to gluten ingestion. The important thing to note is that these patients did not have coeliac disease – however, they were gluten sensitive. Their blood test results are given. The IgG-Gliadin is the most sensitive test. For this particular test, normal values are usually less than 10 units. Similarly, IgA-Gliadin is usually less than 10 units. The tTG (tissue transglutaminase) should be less than 20 units: a high tTG is indicative of coeliac disease.

Ray (36 years)

IgG-gliadin 30   IgA-gliadin 13   tTG 8
Biopsy: not done
Headaches. A family who is gluten-sensitive.

Q. You said that gluten causes your headaches:
Ray said: "Yes! I used to get a lot of headaches. There seemed to be no real reason for it. My kids ended up with a gluten intolerance or a sensitivity. So I went on a gluten-free diet too. I started to reduce the gluten in my diet. Since then, my headaches have greatly reduced. I do know that, if I have gluten to any high degree, within 24–48 hours I have very severe headaches back again."

"A couple of slices of bread gives me headaches. I can have a couple of slices of bread over a couple of days and this brings them on. I also notice that eating a lot of little gluten things adds up to give me the same effect."

Q. How long does it take for the headaches to go?
"It takes about 7–8 hours for this sort of headache to go. I can hit them with three paracaetamol tablets every 4 hours and that takes the top off it. But it is still there a couple of days later. It feels like a bruise on my head, like a distant headache. Even though I have the headache on one day, even the next day it just feels like a massive bruise. It feels like the pains have gone but the pressure or whatever is still there. The shadow is left. It takes a while to go."

Q. Are you convinced that gluten causes these headaches?
"Yes. I am certain. Yes, it certainly has a large affect on them."

James *(8 years)*

IgG-Gliadin 34   IgA-gliadin 7   tTG not done
EMA negative   Biopsy: not done.

Q. Can you tell me about your headaches?
James said: "When I eat gluten, I usually start off getting headaches or stomach pains. Mostly I get the headaches. They usually get worser and worser. But when I get the headache and the stomach pains together, they start going back. It's like the waves going up and down, they go up and then down, up and then down."

Q. How quickly do the headaches come on?
"They come slowly, until they get to a certain level – usually a couple of hours. It takes a while for them to go away. It really depends. Usually it's about five hours, but sometimes by the next day."

Q. How do you feel about being gluten-free?
"If I could have bread I wouldn't be so annoyed. But yeah, it's not that bad because I have found some foods that are a bit like some of the old ones. It depends what everyone else in the family is eating. Sometimes if they are having mince pies and bread, it is difficult. Sometimes it is hard when they are teasing me!"

Rowan *(34 years)*

Blood tests: not done   Biopsy: not done
Gluten-free because his wife and son were on a gluten-free diet.

Rowan said: "My headaches are now so much better controlled. I was having migraines once a week and I would need to take some paracaetamol or even lie down. But sometimes this didn't control it. However, since I have been gluten-free. I would now only have migraines once every three or four weeks. I used to have them every week! Now I notice that they mostly come on when I am more tired and stressed. When I was on gluten these migraines just came out of the blue. It's such a relief to be able to control them now. Thank goodness for this diagnosis!"

7. Damaged nerves and stunted growth

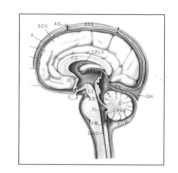

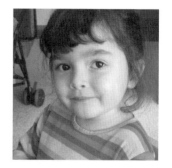

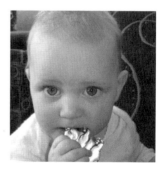

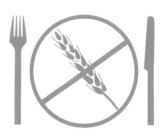

Nerve damage and stunted growth

Nerve damage - Neuropathy

Neuropathy is when the nerves of your body get damaged. There are nerves running throughout your body. The nerves, which connect your brain up to your skin and muscles, are called the peripheral nerves. This peripheral nerve network is linked to your conscious mind.

You have another set of nerves which fans out to connect your brain up with all of your internal organs – this part of the nervous system is called the "autonomic nervous system" which responds to your *unconscious* mind and your emotions (see the diagram in Chapter 4). I regularly see children who have been diagnosed as having a neurological condition, but turn out to have coeliac disease or a gluten-sensitivity. In my opinion, all children (and adults) who have any neurological problems should have a blood test for their gluten and coeliac antibody levels.

An underlying nutritional deficiency is an unlikely explanation for these neuromuscular disorders. There are a number of arguments for this:

o   Many of the neuromuscular disorders which are described in association with coeliac disease and gluten-sensitivity have an inflammatory or autoimmune basis which cannot be simply generated by food deficiencies.

o   Many neurological disorders are seen in the complete absence of any gastro-intestinal disorder.

o   Many people with gluten related neuropathy have no physical or biochemical evidence of malabsorption or nutritional deficiency.

Peripheral neuropathy

Again, with looking through the narrow window of coeliac disease, when looked for carefully, up to 49% of adults with coeliac disease have evidence of a peripheral neuropathy (Cicarelli, 2003). The most common form of neuropathy has been the loss of feelings or a change in sensation felt in the skin. It is usually found in the hands and feet. In a group of 20 patients with neuropathy and confirmed coeliac disease, there were nine patients who had complained of their *sensory* symptoms before the diagnosis of coeliac disease had been made (Chin, 2003).

Gluten can cause loss of feeling

Motor neuropathy

In addition to these sensory disturbances, the *motor* nerves can also be affected. The motor nerves are the nerves that work your muscles which are attached to your bones. They give you the ability to move.

Gluten can cause weakness

So when you get a motor neuropathy you will be weak and not be able to move very well. You will tire very easily. This damage is called a motor neuropathy. Serious damage can be detected in the motor nerves by a technique called electrophysiologic studies. Electrodes are placed over the nerve which is then stimulated by a tiny electric shock. The speed of the nerve conduction can be measured. If the nerve electricity is travelling abnormally slowly, then this is evidence that the nerve has been damaged.

But early on in this condition, the nerve might not be damaged enough to cause a slowing of the current. Of interest, one study (Chin 2003) reported a group of 400 patients who had a neuropathy but had *normal* electrophysiologic studies. They were all investigated for coeliac disease which was found in 8% of them. This is ten times the number that was expected – as the incidence of coeliac disease is about one in one hundred in the population at large.

The reports on the effect of a gluten-free diet on peripheral neuropathy associated with coeliac disease are conflicting. Some studies have reported that a gluten-free diet is effective (Kaplan, 1988; Polizzi, 2000). However, others have found that the neuropathy symptoms have persisted despite an adequate gluten-free diet (Luostarinen, 2003). Again, it is likely that the more chronic and established the disease, the less likely it is to respond to a gluten-free diet. I think this is why children respond so well. Most of the studies are in grown-ups!

Developmental delay

This story is about Oliver. His parents brought him to see me for another opinion when he was 3 years old. He was sent to see me for assessment of his "developmental delay". His parents were naturally very concerned about him. He had already been seen at the "early intervention" program. But he was not making much headway. He had been seen by the physiotherapists who were giving him lots of exercises to do – but this was having no benefit.

When I saw him I was taken aback. I was surprised that he had been seen by so many health professionals, but he looked pale and sick. He had a huge pot tummy. He was incredibly weak. His weakness was from a gluten induced myopathy that quickly recovered once he was gluten-free. He had coeliac disease. His mother tells some of his story:

Oliver (4 years)

IgG-gliadin 157   IgA-gliadin 117   tTG 135
Biopsy: severe villous atrophy (coeliac disease)
Muscle weakness (myopathy), slow development.
Gastric reflux, diarrhoea, vomiting, abdominal pain.

Not developing properly

Mum said: "By 18 months I was a little concerned as I realised that Oliver was saying less than he had been at 12 months. Then, between 18 months and 2 years, he didn't put on any weight. I was reassured by his visiting child health nurse. However, it was during this time that Oliver began to have bouts of diarrhoea and then he started to vomit regularly. I had a growing sense that something wasn't right with Oliver."

Vomiting, diarrhoea, sore tummy and fussy eating

"Then, at 2½ years, after a few more bouts of vomiting and/or diarrhoea (that seemed to come every 3 or so weeks), I took him to see a locum who suggested that maybe Oliver was lactose intolerant. We went lactose-free and the vomiting stopped. But by now, he was often complaining of a sore tummy and the diarrhoea continued. Oliver had also become steadily more fussy with his diet. The things he wouldn't eat were quite unusual for a child. For example, he stopped eating biscuits, ice cream cones and toast. If we gave him an iced bun he'd only eat the icing. I went back to the doctor at 2 years 10 months and asked to see a specialist."

Coeliac disease diagnosed

"Oliver by this stage was not well. He was seriously anaemic, had poor muscle tone, and had a bloated stomach. He was malnourished. I cried as I left Dr Ford's office because I felt so stupid for not pushing for action earlier. I had allowed my GP and health nurse to reassure me all that time, despite as a mother I had felt for a long time that something was wrong. I felt Oliver's health had been seriously compromised because I hadn't trusted my instincts. Dr

Ford basically diagnosed coeliac disease on this first visit. A blood test and subsequent endoscopy confirmed this. I worried about the consequences that his serious lack of iron may have had on his brain development."

An urgent endoscopy
"Oliver was gluten-free from the time I left the office that day. When Dr Ford called with the blood test results he said that, ordinarily, a patient should stay on a gluten containing diet until the endoscopy. But because Oliver was so sick, he should immediately go off gluten. The endoscopy showed severe villus atrophy – the confirmation of coeliac disease."

His personality changed
"Off gluten Oliver became much more external. Instead of what I perceived as a child who was content within himself, suddenly we had a child who was much more interested in the outside world, and he began to notice people outside himself. He quickly became strong again and caught up with all of those milestones that were lagging behind."

We quickly coped with gluten-free
"Oliver put on 6kgs in his first 6 months on a gluten-free diet. We didn't have too many difficulties with the diet itself. It was however a big learning curve. I did some research on the internet. We saw a dietician. We joined the Coeliac Society. In the early stages we read a lot of labels. We couldn't believe how many things contained gluten. It was frustrating and upsetting. I was upset that Oliver would never be able to drink beer!"

He is now happy and content. What a relief!
"Oliver has been fantastic about his gluten-free diet. He seems to totally accept that he cannot eat some foods. For a time, however, he thought that he would be able to eat these foods when he was big like his big brother. We refer to gluten-free foods as gluten-free or

"special". We have explained that his tummy is special and that it only likes special foods. It has become even easier since his Dad has gone gluten-free (he is not coeliac but feels much better for it). He now has an ally. His baby sister is also gluten-free in the meantime. It's such a relief to have my son healthy and strong again."

Autonomic neuropathy

Your autonomic nervous system takes care of your vital day-to-day body functions that you never have to think about. This system keeps going day and night. It keeps you breathing, keeps your heart pumping, and keeps your gut working faultlessly. Although it is not under your conscious control, it is strongly influenced by your emotions. Control of your swallowing, your stomach emptying, the flow of food through your intestines, and your colonic movements are all mediated through this system.

There is now lots of evidence of upper-gut motor abnormalities in many people with coeliac disease. This topic has been carefully researched (Usai, 1977) in an investigation of upper-gut motor activity in 30 coeliac patients. They then explored the role played by the autonomic nervous system in these motility disturbances.

Autonomic system malfunctions in most coeliacs

They found oesophageal motor abnormalities in half of their patients. Abnormal oesophageal acid studies (pH-probes) were abnormal in 30%. Delayed gastric emptying was documented in 50%. In total, 75% of coeliac patients were shown to have some sort of gastro-intestinal motility alterations. Tests of autonomic dysfunction were positive in 45% of these patients. This indicated that a gluten autonomic neuropathy was playing a role in their reflux.

105

Ataxia

Ataxia is the word for when you feel wobbly or if you have an unsteady gait or walk. It is a loss of coordination. Ataxia can be due to damage of the cerebellum. The cerebellum looks like a wrinkled clenched fist of tissue at the back of your brain. Your cerebellum coordinates your body movements. Your cerebellum is also involved in the learning of repeated movements. For example, when you catch a ball, or balance on one leg, or use the computer keyboard – when you are carrying out these learned repetitive movements, then you are training your cerebellum.

Gluten can make you wobbly

Movement control

This cerebellum co-ordination of your body movement is achieved by collecting information from all parts of your body. This information of awareness about the position of your body comes hurtling in from all of your nerve sensors (limb position, balance information, speed, and what you can see). Eventually, this stream of information can help you do things like learn how to ride a bike without falling over. And then, magically, your cerebellum remembers this set of instructions, forever.

Some of the symptoms that are associated with damage to the cerebellum or the nervous tracts leading to it are:
o   Ataxia (difficulty in coordinating movements)
o   Tremors
o   Loss of balance, vertigo, and dizziness
o   Muscle weakness
o   Difficulty in performing rapid alternating movements
o   Loss of postural tone.

Gluten ataxia

There is much evidence that gluten is the culprit in causing these symptoms in many people. Gluten can impair the function of the cerebellum. It was forty years ago that the first cases of ataxia that were linked to coeliac disease were reported (Cooke and Smith, 1966). They wrote about a group of 16 patients with coeliac disease who also had gait ataxia and peripheral neuropathy. They demonstrated that these patients had cerebellar dysfunction.

Gluten impairs function of the cerebellum

Many others have subsequently shown that cerebellar ataxia, and indeed many other neurological syndromes, may be part of the presenting symptoms of coeliac disease. In one such study, a group of patients with cerebellar ataxia (of unknown cause) were investigated by small bowel biopsy: 16% (4 of 25) were found to have coeliac disease (Pellecchi, 1999).

Gluten the troublemaker

The next step in my reasoning is this: gluten may be the troublemaker in the brain *without* the need to be associated with coeliac disease. This is now called gluten-sensitivity. Hadjivassiliou (1999) has put it like this: "It remains controversial whether gluten-sensitivity (a state of heightened immunologic responsiveness to ingested gluten) without intestinal involvement should be considered the cause of cerebellar degeneration in ataxia of otherwise unknown cause." Various studies have found that the prevalence of positive IgG-gliadin antibodies in ataxia (of unknown cause) has varied between 0–41%. However, raised IgG-gliadin antibodies are found more frequently in ataxia (30%) than in the general population (8–12%). This is excellent evidence for a causal association between cerebellar degeneration and gluten-sensitivity.

Gluten-driven brain inflammation

The mechanism of how this damage is caused is still uncertain. It also is controversial whether the IgG-gliadin antibodies might directly interact with the nervous system. However, there are some case histories which provide evidence that the gluten damage is from inflammatory disease.

Gluten reactions can be inflammatory

For example, a patient described in this following case report demonstrates the gluten-driven inflammation (Ghezzi, 1997). A patient with both coeliac disease and progressive brain symptoms (suggesting brainstem and cerebellar involvement) had a series of MRI brain scans. The first examination showed multiple brain lesions. Soon after, a large cerebellar lesion appeared, and then this was followed by severe cerebellar atrophy. The presence of structural neuronal damage was confirmed by another type of brain scan (proton MR spectroscopy and magnetization transfer imaging). The MRI results and spinal fluid tests suggested that these neurological complications were more likely due to an inflammatory process.

Evidence of nerve damage

There are some very sensitive cells in the cerebellum (the part of the brain responsible for coordination). They are called "Purkinje cells" and function as the output neurons of the cerebellum. These are the cells that appear to be most susceptible to damage in patients with this gluten-ataxia. Recent study results have shown that patients with gluten-ataxia have antibodies against these Purkinje cells.

Gluten antibodies cross-react with brain cells

Additionally, they found that antibodies directed against gluten (the IgG-gliadin antibodies) actually cross-react with Purkinje cells (Hadjivassiliou). To explain, this means that although the initial immune reaction was mounted against the gluten protein, by chance, this antibody also reacted to the Purkinje nerve cells. This is a fatal attraction and causes subsequent nerve damage in the cerebellum.

Neurological dysfunction of unknown cause

In medicine, the causes of many illnesses are unknown. In the brain areas, the phrase used to describe such unknown diseases is "neurological dysfunction of obscure aetiology." When such a group of patients was investigated for gluten reactions, a high prevalence of antigliadin antibodies (57%) was found in their blood compared with two control groups (5–27%). But only a third of these patients had histological evidence of coeliac disease.

High IgG-gliadin antibodies in brain dysfunction

The conclusion drawn was that the remaining two thirds (65%) had gluten-sensitivity. The target organ in this case was the cerebellum or the peripheral nerves.

Finally, both the ataxia (from cerebellar damage) and the neuropathy are often reversible on a strict gluten-free diet. The authors (Hadjivassiliou 1998) went on to say, "These results strengthen our contention that eliminating these antibodies through strict adherence to a gluten-free diet may have important therapeutic implications for patients with gluten ataxia." Here the focus is on antibody reduction rather than just the elimination of gluten. Surely there is a strong case for investigating for gluten-sensitivity in *all* patients with any neurological dysfunction.

Epilepsy

Epilepsy is a brain condition. It is the spontaneous discharge of electrical activity in the brain. This causes a sudden change in behaviour or motor activity. The symptoms and signs depend upon where in the brain this abnormal activity is occurring. In the general population, about one in every fifty people has some sort of experience of epileptic seizures. Yet again, there is an association between coeliac disease and epilepsy, although this does not seem to be very strong. A higher prevalence of epilepsy (3.5–5.5%) has been reported in patients with coeliac disease compared with controls (2%). Also, high IgG-gliadin antibody levels are more prevalent in patients with primary generalized epilepsy (19.6%) than in the reference population (10.6%) (Ranua, 2005).

Gluten-sensitivity is linked to epilepsy

In addition, the specific condition "bilateral occipital cerebral calcification and seizures" has been more strongly associated with coeliac disease (Visakorpi, 1970). However, this syndrome seems to be rare. In one study (Fois, 1994), 783 children who presented with seizures were investigated for coeliac disease: there were nine children discovered with partial and/or grand mal seizures. Of these, only three (0.3%) had cerebral calcification.

The effect of a gluten-free diet on epilepsy control in coeliac disease has been variable. In most patients the beneficial effects of the diet have been reported in terms of better seizure control and a decrease in the amounts of antiepileptic medications – but not the resolution of their seizures. Perhaps, the earlier the diagnosis and treatment with a gluten-free diet, the better the outcome. Again, all children with epilepsy should be investigated for evidence of gluten-sensitivity.

Stunted Growth

Poor growth is very commonly found in children who are sensitive to gluten. My studies have found that about a quarter of all children who react to gluten show some degree of slowing in their height growth.

Gluten interferes with growth hormone action

Poor growth is seen even more frequently in those with established coeliac disease. In this situation, their poor nutrition will be compounding the problem. But the evidence is mounting that these children's growth failure is more to do with growth hormone malfunction than with any associated malabsorption.

Growth hormone suppression

Growth hormone is crucial for the maintenance of *height* growth. Growth hormone is manufactured in the centre of your brain, in a place called the pituitary gland. Growth hormone gets released in surges when you are stressed and when you are sleeping.

Gluten puts a break on growth

It turns out that gluten can cause suppression of this growth hormone release. This means that although the child has the capacity to produce this growth hormone, the body cannot make enough of it because it is stopped by gluten. When I explain this to parents, I say that gluten acts like a break on growth. Take the child off gluten and the child begins to grow again. Usually this bounce back starts within a few months, but sometimes it can take a little longer.

The growth hormone evidence

This evidence comes from a number of studies. Federico (1997) studied 14 children with coeliac disease. He carried out very detailed growth hormone tests both before and after these children had been on a gluten-free diet for six months.

Before treatment with a gluten-free diet, most of these children had abnormal measurements for most of their growth hormone tests. The researchers concluded that coeliac children had *multiple* alterations in their growth hormone system during the time when they were suffering from the ill-effects of their coeliac disease.

Gluten upsets growth hormone function

However, after the six month period on a gluten-free diet, they found that these growth hormone abnormalities had disappeared. Of great importance, the actual height measurements improved significantly in these children after they had been on the diet. Excitingly, those with the most severe growth hormone suppression grew the best after gluten had been removed.

Children grow well off gluten

Another large set of studies was carried out to assess the occurrence of growth hormone deficiency in patients with coeliac disease. It showed similar findings (Bozzola, 2005). This study was based on a group of 1066 children diagnosed with short stature. All of these children were tested for coeliac disease using the endomysial antibody (EMA) test. Those with a positive test then had an intestinal biopsy. Of these 1066 short children, about a fifth (210, 19.7%) had growth hormone deficiency. Only 12 were diagnosed as having coeliac disease.

The study then only focused on these 12 children with coeliac disease. Nine of these children showed a good growth rate, catching up after the first year of a gluten-free diet. But the other three had no catch-up growth. A careful endocrinological investigation showed that they had a persistent growth hormone deficiency. Subsequent treatment with growth hormone replacement therapy (associated with a continued gluten-free diet) eventually led to an increased growth rate.

So they concluded that growth hormone secretion should be evaluated in coeliac patients who show no catch-up growth after a period on a gluten-free diet. They might need extra growth hormone therapy.

Some coeliacs are growth hormone deficient

Gluten-sensitivity and poor growth

The implication of the above studies is that gluten-sensitivity, rather than the nutritional deficiency, is the cause of the growth hormone suppression. Thus my observations extend the problem.

The traditional view in the investigation of short stature is to look for coeliac disease. If small bowel damage is not found, then any reaction to gluten is dismissed. I think that this is wrong.

My evidence is that there are many more children who are gluten-sensitive than those who are found to have coeliac disease. Of these gluten-sensitive children, about a fifth have poor growth. This can usually be reversed when they go on a gluten-free diet.

Test all short children

I argue that all children who are small (for either height or weight) should be tested both for coeliac disease and for gluten-sensitivity. This means looking for a raised IgG-gliadin antibody level as well as for tissue-damage antibodies (tTG).

Test all children who are short

In addition, as the susceptibility to gluten reactions seems to be largely genetic, even when short stature appears to be a family trait, the possibility that gluten could be an underlying cause in all family members needs to be considered.

The next facet of gluten-sensitivity to be examined is disturbances in mood and behaviour.

8. Mood and behaviour

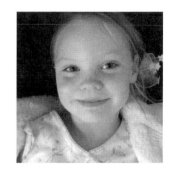

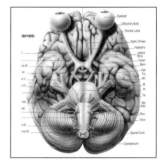

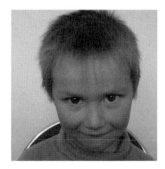

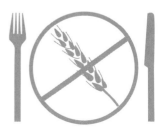

Mood and behaviour

In my experience, mood and behaviour problems are amongst the most common symptoms of gluten-sensitivity. However, the age old question arises again: "What is normal?"

So many people are tired, they lack energy and they are moody. Therefore, these attributes are considered "normal". Some people are just like that! Then add the hassles and responsibilities of caring for little children! Many people think that life is exhausting.

The phases of childhood also embody expected behaviour problems. We label the preschool and toddler age group as the "terrible twos", the "tiresome threes" and the "fearsome fours". And then there are the teenagers. I suspect that a lot of these adverse and difficult behaviours are driven by reactions to gluten.

These apparently "normal" symptoms have been noted in a recent study on the prevalence of coeliac disease (Hoffenberg 2004). The parents of apparently "asymptomatic" children were interviewed as part of a population study to identify those with coeliac disease. They found many children who had positive tests for coeliac disease also had irritability, lethargy, abdominal distention, gas, and poor weight gains.

Unfortunately, many people do not know what it feels like to be "normal". I now present a series of people who have had symptoms that have been eventually attributed to gluten-sensitivity. In my opinion these people have been suffering from neurological or brain disturbances, caused by gluten. They subsequently recovered on a gluten-free diet. Improved nutrition, a boost in iron and zinc levels, and a happy tummy will also contribute to their improved sense of wellbeing.

The best way that I can tell you about the mood and behaviour problems is to let people tell their own stories. I have either interviewed people or asked them to write down their own stories. You can make your own conclusions. Again, a normal IgG-gliadin antibody level is below 10 units.

Lethargy, low energy

The world seems to be full of people who are worn out, tired and exhausted. People who are desperately seeking the secret of finding energy. Gluten-sensitivity saps people of energy. Anyone who feels sick and tired should get a gluten blood test.

Lochlainn (9 years)

IgG-gliadin 111   IgA-gliadin 22   tTG 13
Biopsy: not done.

This boy, Lochie, thought that he was "normal". But he was lethargic, he was slowing down at school. He couldn't be bothered to work. He lacked energy.

Lochie said: "Hi! My name is Lochie. I went to see the doctor with my brother Mac. Dr Ford said that I might have the same thing as my brother and I should be tested. I am nine years old."

Reflux and milk allergy as a baby
"When I was a baby my mother said that I had silent reflux and had to take medicine to be able to eat or drink. I couldn't have dairy or soy for a long time. Eventually I grew out of it and could have some dairy."

"I love food and have always eaten heaps! I am very clever and love school. I never get into trouble at school like my brother and I win awards for academic stuff every year. I am fast too – I won my year's duathlon."

Anything wrong with me?

"I did not know there was anything wrong with me. When Mum talked to the doctor she said that I had seemed to be losing interest in my work and did not want to go for walks. I have lots of trouble going to the toilet and have to spend ages there, I don't like going because it hurts. I started to get a pot tummy. I had a blood test and the levels for gluten were very high."

Embarrassed going gluten-free

"I stopped eating gluten and find it a bit embarrassing. I didn't want to go to camp because I don't want to eat food that is different from everyone else. Mum makes us really nice food, and you can buy a lot of stuff in the shops now. Some of the new stuff she makes doesn't work out!"

More energy off gluten

"Since I have been gluten-free my pot tummy has disappeared. I am sort of happy to be gluten-free because I have got more energy. I am back to reading chapter books and doing all my homework on Monday nights. I am going to play Soccer starting next month.

But I am sort of sad too because I can't eat a lot of food that I loved. We talk about all the other children who have other disabilities and it makes me think ours isn't too bad. I have problems with coordination and balance. I have only just now learnt to ride my bike. Dr Ford said that this might be to do with gluten too. I am now doing exercises and juggling to try and get things better."

Glenda (27 years)

IgG-gliadin 34   IgA-gliadin 6   tTG 4
Biopsy: not done.
Lazy and lethargic.

Glenda has always been tired and lacked energy. But nothing could be found and so she was just considered to be a lazy person. She is the mother of one of my patients.

Glenda said: "For as long as I can remember, I used to always feel so very tired and had very little energy. As I was growing up my parents often described me as lazy."

Why was I tired all of the time?

"Over the years I have had a variety of medical tests to try and find out the reason for me being so very tired all of the time. Tests for glandular fever, thyroid problems and anaemia all came back negative. Also, I had always had problems passing bowel motions."

"It wasn't until I was visiting my son's paediatrician, for something that I thought had nothing to do with me at all, that I began to get some answers. I was five months pregnant with my second child when, through blood tests ordered by my son's paediatrician, I discovered that I might be gluten-sensitive. The paediatrician wanted my son to try a gluten-free diet – so I thought that I might as well give it a try too."

Absolutely fantastic! So much more energy!

"Within two weeks I was feeling absolutely fantastic! I could not ever remember having so much energy – and I was 5 months pregnant. I could stay up until 10.30 pm every night with ease. Previously, I had struggled to stay up to 8.30 pm and in my first pregnancy I was lucky if I was awake at 7.30 pm. My bowel motions also become much easier to pass."

"After I had been gluten-free for three weeks I decide to test the theory. I ate some food containing gluten. Within hours my stomach was uncomfortable. I developed diarrhoea, had a really sore tongue and generally felt pretty awful. So that was enough proof for me that gluten was not good for my body."

Gluten-free is inconvenient

"The hardest thing about going gluten-free is the inconvenience of it. I now have to go to three separate supermarkets as they all stock different gluten-free foods. Grocery shopping also takes a lot longer as I read the labels on just about everything before I buy it. Also, the easy option of getting take-a-ways for dinner is pretty much gone."

"However, the rest of the world seems to be coming more aware: there are so many more gluten-free products available now compared with even six months ago. Buying gluten-free products is much more expensive than buying the gluten-containing equivalent."

"However, the expense of the gluten-free food isn't too much to pay to have so much energy and not to feel exhausted all of the time. I almost feel normal!!"

Sarah (32 years)

IgG-gliadin 56   IgA-gliadin 14   tTG 62
Biopsy: normal small bowel, low disaccharidases, oesophagitis.

Tired, exhausted, low energy.
Difficult to think clearly.

Sarah was a busy mum who felt completely exhausted all of the time. She was also troubled with depression. She has two children who have recently been diagnosed with gluten-sensitivity.

Q. When you have gluten, how quickly does it affect you?
Sarah said: "Yes. When I have gluten it affects me within a couple of hours. I feel very very tired."

"I feel so tired that I have to go to sleep. I feel that tired. I feel I want to sleep all the time. It is a time you don't get over. It is a time which even if you have a sleep, it still doesn't make any difference. You still wake up tired!"

Q. How much gluten causes you trouble?
"I am so careful with what I eat. I just don't want to feel sick again. I have been out to restaurants and must have eaten some gluten without me knowing it. So I don't think it takes a lot to make me feel so tired and exhausted. I know because I always check."

"Also the gluten can affect how you are thinking. When I have had gluten, my thinking goes all blurry. When I am not on gluten, I can think a lot more clearly. But when I try and think with the gluten, it is all of a blur. It is much more hard work."

121

Leigh (35 years)

IgG-gliadin 24   IgA-gliadin 4   tTG 6
Biopsy: not done.

Irritable, tired, low energy.
Great improvement gluten-free.

Leigh is another mum who gets extreme tiredness with the ingestion of small amounts of gluten. Going gluten-free has been a life-saver for her.

Leigh said: "Since finding out I was gluten sensitive, my overall well-being has improved considerably. There are still days, however, where I wake up wondering what I have eaten the day before that has made me feel so yuk. On these days, I feel like I am dragging around a load of bricks. Even the smallest tasks feel like major battles. I am irritable and tired, and feel like collapsing on the couch to do nothing."

"By the afternoon on these days, between 3–6 pm, my mood changes, and I can feel the lethargy floating away. Then I feel able to achieve everything that had seemed so challenging earlier."

"To me, it feels as though whatever is affecting me has been broken down by my body by the afternoon, or that the food I have eaten that day, has diluted the effect."

"Of course, living with a two-year old, and being pregnant, may have something to do with it also!"

James (31 years)

IgG-gliadin 84   IgA-gliadin 18   tTG 16
Biopsy: not done.
Multiple Sclerosis.

James had a diagnosis of multiple sclerosis. However he is also gluten-sensitive and now feels very much better off gluten. He is now full of energy again. Every person with a neurological problem should be tested for gluten-sensitivity.

James said: "At 21 years of age (when I was working as a car painter), I started to suffer from exhaustion whenever I was in the heat of the sun. My pulse would start to race, but I would recover quickly once in the shade. When at home I noticed that I would regularly forget that I was holding something, and then drop it. I also suffered from light-headedness when in the shower and would often collapse, catching myself before hitting the floor."

Multiple sclerosis diagnosed
"As time went on, I started to experience tingling down the left side of my face and body. This went on for about a week. I was driven home from work one day and put to bed with these symptoms by 10 am. By 12 noon an ambulance was called. I had lost the ability to speak, and the left side of my face was drooping. By 2 pm I had lost the movement and feeling down the left side of my body. I was subjected to a CAT scan, MRI, lumber puncture, and a multitude of blood tests. It took three weeks to regain the use of my left side, and the slur that I had slowly disappeared. About one month later I lost the sight in my right eye. This confirmed the diagnosis of Multiple Sclerosis."

"I have had a 99% recovery, and have managed to prevent further attacks with plenty of rest, a good diet, and the use of a high quality multivitamin, mineral supplement and antioxidant."

Much better gluten-free

"This year I have gone gluten-free after my son was diagnosed with coeliac disease. My blood test showed that I was probably gluten-sensitive showing a very high IgG gliadin antibody level. Within weeks I have noticed that my sinus problem has cleared up. For the first time in 30 years I can breathe easily. My bowel motions are more regular. The re-occurring eczema on my arm has cleared up. My energy levels have increased dramatically (for which my boss is grateful). My mood swings are controllable (for which my boys are grateful). And my memory has improved (for which my wife is grateful)."

"Our entire family has made the decision to be gluten-free. We feel that the positive side effects outweigh the negative. Our diet is much healthier. We have been forced into becoming more aware of what we put into our mouths. Cutting out foods filled with unnecessary additives, preservatives, colourings and flavourings can only be beneficial to our longevity and health. We have also found the food to be much more tasty and enjoyable, possibly due to not feeling ill every time we eat."

Angry

There are so many angry and grumpy people about. Anger is very destructive and leads to poor family relationships and loss of self-esteem. Gluten appears to be an important trigger for angry outbursts in many people. Ben is a good example of this. On gluten he cannot cope. He now recognises that gluten makes him feel angry.

Benjamin (6 years)

IgG-gliadin 25   IgA-gliadin 4   tTG 4
Biopsy: not done.

Ben said: "I got angry on gluten".
Mum said: "Ben was challenged with gluten two days ago. He relapsed. He got very angry, he fought his sister, he hit, he yelled and he burst into crying. He was really, really angry and couldn't cope with anything."

"He really went at his sisters. He was throwing things about when he got cross. He would hit, yell, scream, burst into tears. Crying all the time. He was always just really, really angry and just couldn't cope with anything. When anything went wrong he just couldn't cope with it. He just didn't know how to deal with it."

"Now, after two days he is back on a gluten-free diet. He started on the diet again yesterday. Just two days ago all this terrible behaviour happened. Today, thankfully, has been much much better! No headaches. No funny poos."

Ben said: "We tried normal food for a while, so I went back on gluten. I got angry. For two days on gluten I was not very good. The next day I got really angry. I was always grumpy as well. I am back on my diet and I already feel much better."

Charlotte (3 years)

IgG gliadin 56   IgA gliadin 3   tTG not done
Endomysial antibodies negative.
Biopsy: not done.
Behaviour changes.

Charlotte was angry, cross and difficult. She was irritable, grizzly and grumpy. She was diagnosed as gluten-sensitive when she came to see me because of behaviour problems. As soon as she went onto the gluten-free diet her behaviour changed for the better. Her irritability was being driven by gluten.

A big change off gluten

Mum said: "Charlotte had been gluten-free for the last three months. It had made a big difference to her behaviour. When she first went gluten-free there was a complete change! A complete turn around from her personality. She wasn't so aggressive and so argumentative. She was a much happier child. She got on with her sister and didn't fight and argue. She also now sleeps much, much better. This change in her personality happened within five or six days."

"Perhaps the main thing we have noticed is that she no longer is in pain with sore legs at night. As soon as she went gluten-free her leg pains disappeared. We know when she has had gluten because she complains of pain in the night again."

Q: What happens when she now eats gluten?

Mum said: "She just becomes more difficult to parent. She becomes so independent. She says "I do it myself". You can't help her do anything, she is so independent. She is irritable, grizzly, and grumpy. She fights with her sister, and refuses to do what you say. She will do the opposite just to annoy you. This comes on within a few hours. Then, by the next day she is fine."

Georgia (4 years)

IgG gliadin 70   IgA gliadin 7   tTG 4
Biopsy: not done.

Growly, constipation, abdominal pains, poor eating, and poor sleeping.

Georgia had always been a growly and irritable girl. She was considered a naughty girl. She is now happy and good off gluten. Gluten had been making her cantankerous.

Naughty
Mum said: "Georgia has grandparents who just did not believe me when I said that she got sick with gluten. They just thought that she was just a growly irritable girl."

Happy
"But when we went up to stay with them for Christmas, Georgia had been off gluten for about six months. It was then that they (her grand parents) noticed that she was a happy child and they commented on the absolute difference with her."

"She was happy and running around. She was happy, interacting with people, when before she used to just cry and sit on my knee. She also had constipation and was a bit cantankerous in the past."

She is extremely sensitive to gluten
"And it is only a small amount of gluten that can upset her – for example, just a bite of biscuit. After about an hour, not straight away, she will start getting growly and whingy. Then she starts having stomach problems, stomach cramps. She gets quite upset – maybe growly is the best word. This can last up to a week."

"Georgia gets a personality change within hours of having small amounts of gluten."

Olivia (8 years)

IgG-gliadin 33   IgA-gliadin 7   tTG 5
Biopsy: not done
Headaches, poor concentration, angry and irritable.

Olivia tells us how she feels when eating gluten. Her symptoms take a while to come on. Her school teacher also noticed the changes in her.

Q. What happened when you had a gluten-challenge?
Olivia said: "When I went onto gluten, I had tummy pains, ulcers and headaches. When I went off gluten I got better. I had been off gluten for about six months. I got fed up with being gluten-free. So I decided to break my diet and go back on gluten again."

"I was very pleased at first. For the next three weeks back on gluten I was feeling reasonable – although I had a bit more eczema and a little bit more hay fever. But then I started getting sore tummies again. I had headaches. I got really, really tired and my concentration wasn't very good. I would go off and start doing other things and get really tired."

Q. What happened at school?
"I'd start thinking about other things, not concentrating. And then I would go back to my desk and then I would be thinking "how am I supposed to do this?" and I would realise that I hadn't been listening. So, I would have to ask the teacher how to do it all over again. It was really hard. I would get really tired when I got home and I would sometimes get really angry and shout sometimes. I got really grumpy."

Q. How did you sleep?
"In the weekends I would be able to get up really early, but then when I had to go back to school on Monday I would never get up. I wouldn't want to get up. So basically, it was the opposite way than it should be."

Mother adds: "Olivia has been diagnosed as dyslexic and she has tutoring once a week for an hour. She gets taken out of class and she has a special teacher to tutor her. The tutor herself has got coeliac disease and she noticed a big difference in Olivia's concentration between when she was gluten-free and when she went back onto gluten. She saw a marked decline in her concentration ability during the gluten challenge. Thank goodness that she is getting better again. I have found this all very interesting. It is hard to believe that gluten could so badly affect her brain."

Joshua (4 years)

IgG-gliadin 129   IgA-gliadin 12   tTG 4
Biopsy: not done
He gets so angry with gluten!

Joshua is also very sensitive to gluten. Within a few minutes a behavioural change is seen. He gets into a very angry mood. He is so much better when off gluten. It is amazing.

Q: What is your first sign of any gluten in his diet?
Mum said: "If he tasted gluten, not even in a meal but on play dough, he gets very angry, totally behavioural. He becomes unruly. From there, then the obvious things are rashes on his face and he gets a bloated tummy very quickly – within the day."

Q: How quickly does he get angry?
"Within minutes. With just the play dough at kindergarten. He is only just playing with it and then his hands go into his mouth. He doesn't even have to eat the play dough, but then the rash starts around the mouth and the behaviour goes downhill. He comes out in a really angry mood."

ADHD and learning problems

Attention Deficit Hyperactivity Disorder (ADHD) and learning disabilities have only recently been recognised as being associated with coeliac disease (Zelnik, 2004). However, my work shows that gluten-sensitivity is also clearly related to these problems.

I constantly see children who are not doing well at school. They have difficulty concentrating in the classroom. They are impulsive, fidgety and sometimes defiant. Others are tired and have difficulty understanding what is being taught. They get confused. They are often better off with individual tuition rather than in a class full of other children. I have now recognised that many of these children are reacting to the gluten in their diets. When they eventually go gluten-free, within only a few weeks, they begin to settle down at school and their school work vastly improves. Frequently, their teacher spontaneously remarks on their sudden unexpected progress.

This dramatic improvement is likely to be due to a combination of nutritional, immunologic, and inflammatory factors – each of which is playing an important role. Improvement in iron levels and their feeling of increased well being will help them at school. Also the absence of tummy pains and lethargy will help.

However, as you will read, when these children later have gluten infringements, even tiny amounts of gluten then seem to trigger their behaviour and learning problems again. I am now absolutely convinced that the ingestion of gluten causes major behavioural harm to vast numbers of children and adults.

One of the shocking truths about gluten is that this phenomenon is currently almost unrecognised.

Simon (10 years)

IgG-gliadin 55   IgA-gliadin 8   tTG 16
Biopsy: not done.
Lethargy and learning problems.

Simon was brought to see me because of his behaviour issues. He was a challenging and defiant. He was failing at school and his parents were very concerned. He got completely better by simply going on a gluten-free diet. Gluten was causing all of his problems.

We thought he was a lazy child
Mum said: "Simon has suffered from a lot of stomach pains, lethargy, and allergies from different foods. He also had many learning problems. As parents, we thought he was a lazy child as he would always take so long to do things, if at all."

His learning has improved so much
"Simon has been gluten-free for nearly five months now. We could notice a difference almost straight away. His learning improved so much that he was eligible for a high achiever class at his school."

So much more energy
"His energy levels have increased and he is really enjoying his love of sport. He can now last a game of hockey without wanting and needing to come off the field. Simon's spirit has returned and he is the bright, funny and lovable child that he used to be. Now, when Simon has gluten, we can see the difference immediately. It affects his sleeping – he sleep-talks and he is very restless. His energy levels drop considerably and I feel that with continued use of gluten in his diet the other symptoms would rear their ugly heads."

He is so much better!
"We do not want to go down that road again. It is very hard for Simon to be gluten-free but even he realised that he feels much, much better."

Mac (7 years)

IgG-gliadin 82   IgA-gliadin 13   tTG 4
Biopsy: not done.
An ADHD story.

Mac came to see me for diagnosis and management of his apparent ADHD. He also had tummy pains that triggered off the blood tests for gluten. He has made a remarkable recovery on a gluten-free diet.

Lots of food allergies

Mac said: "Hello my name is Mac. I am seven years old. When I was a baby I was very sick. I had gastric reflux and lots of allergies. I could not have milk, eggs, soy, peanuts and had to have special milk from the hospital after Mum stopped breast feeding me."

I was naughty

"I was very naughty when I was a toddler – I hurt people and frightened them. I did not mean to do it. I found it hard to concentrate and I used to run away a lot. I had a special place under the spare bed where I used to hide with my toys. I love chocolate."

"Mum and Dad took me to lots of doctors and they just said I was an unusual wee boy. They said that I might need to be treated with ADHD medications. Mum used positive reinforcement and things were still a bit sad at school. Dad took me to the hospital to get grommets to see if it was my hearing that was making me cross."

I couldn't concentrate

"When I started school, I was in trouble every day – I couldn't concentrate on work and used to annoy people or go and hide under my desk when my teachers growled at me. I always had diarrhoea and a sore tummy. Mum and Dad knew there was something wrong because they could see in my eyes that I didn't mean to be bad. They said that I was really a kind and special boy."

I'm top of the class off gluten

"Mum took me to see Dr Rodney Ford last year after I got really sick. I had a really sore tummy for weeks and Mum thought it might be because of gluten. We all went to see the special doctor. A blood test showed that I was being made sick by gluten. I felt better really quickly after I stopped eating gluten. I hardly ever get into trouble at school any more. I sometimes still do stuff without thinking and get into trouble. I have a really nice teacher this year. I got the top of my class in maths this year and got a special certificate."

I can read and spell now

"I won the cross country as I can run really fast. I read at level purple which is great and I can spell words like 'children'. My tummy still hurts sometimes and I get a headache sometimes if I eat gluten by accident or on purpose. My brother was made gluten-free a couple of weeks after me so it isn't too bad. I have my own friends now and they want to come over to my place and play. I miss McDonalds and some other stuff."

I love school now

"I love school now and I am going to play rugby for the Harlequins, Crusaders and then be an All Black."

Kara-Leigh (10 years)

IgG-gliadin 89   IgA-gliadin 6   tTG 3
Biopsy: not done.

Symptoms of losing weight, ADD (Attention Deficit Disorder).
Treated with Ritalin for the prior 18 months.

Kara had been on methylphenidate (Ritalin) for over a year. She came to see me because of losing weight and difficulty with her behaviour management. Blood tests showed that she was gluten-sensitive. She was able to come off Ritalin. At last she is progressing at school.

Mum said: "How beautiful she is now that she has been off gluten for three months. She was on Ritalin. She is no longer on Ritalin. Here is what happened at the school interview. She had been on her gluten-free diet for about 10 weeks. Her teacher said that she had become more settled, and her school work had improved."

"At the beginning of the year, one of her projects was just basically a whole lot of scribble. But last week she did another project and it was just amazing the difference. It was well completed and well thought out. She had put a lot of effort into it. The teacher can't get over the difference in her since the stopping of the Ritalin and going on the gluten-free diet."

Del (47 years)

IgG-gliadin 4   IgA-gliadin 4   tTG 12
(Blood tests done while she was on strict gluten-free diet)
Biopsy: not done.

Q. What happens when you have gluten?
Del said: "Last week, I had some gluten late morning. I was tempted by a biscuit! I didn't have much work to do and I came home. It takes me a while to realise that my symptoms must be due to gluten. I get the first symptoms in my head."

"After a few hours I feel really tired and a bit borderline confusion – you know, a bit muddley. And then it peaks and then it takes me a while to understand what is happening to me. And then I think – I must have had some gluten. The last time this happened to me I think it was from the gluten in some corned beef. I get "a coming down with it feeling". After about four hours I just can't do anything and feel tired for the rest of the day. I also get double vision when I have gluten – a sort of blurry feeling".

Autism

Autism is a common developmental disorder of early childhood. It was found in about one in every thousand children. However, many more children are now being diagnosed. This big increase in diagnosis is due to a combination of increasing numbers and better recognition of the problem. Autism is characterised by impairment in social interaction and communication. There is an absence of speech in about half of these children. They seem distant and hard to connect with. They may scream and be incredibly disruptive. There are a number of typical behaviours that these autistic children display: hand flapping, spinning, body rocking, insistence on sameness, resistance to change.

Although the underlying cause of autism remains unclear, evidence of a genetic contribution is based on studies showing high concordance in monozygotic twins. Also, autism can be found with the genetic disorders of fragile X syndrome and tuberous sclerosis.

The role of gluten-sensitivity in autism is seen as tenuous. It is based on the leaky-gut hypothesis. This is an abnormality in the intestinal mucosa which allows the absorption of partially digested food proteins such as gluten and casein. This enhanced absorption then results in an excessive intake of short peptides. These peptides then provoke an immune reaction. They also act as exorphins that directly affect the nervous system. A direct association between coeliac disease and autism has not been established. However, behavioural improvement in autistic children on a gluten-free and casein-free diet has been reported by some groups – but not in others. In my experience, many of the autistic children that I have managed have substantially improved on a gluten-free and casein free diet. Whole books have been written on this subject, so I will leave further speculation to these other authors.

Depression

There is no question that untreated coeliac disease can lead to serious behavioural disorders. The big question that I am examining is whether this is due to brain and nerve damage from gluten. Depression and other psychiatric symptoms are reported as common complications of coeliac disease. These problems affect about a third of coeliac patients. The symptoms include tiredness, apathy, irritability, mood changes, feeling down, excessive anxiety, and irritability. Exhaustion is frequently stated.

There are all sorts of ideas that have been put forward to explain the mechanisms of depression. Malabsorption and nutritional deficiencies (especially of vitamin B6 and tryptophan) are favourite candidates. Decreased blood levels of tryptophan have been demonstrated in coeliac disease. Also, decreased cerebrospinal fluid levels of serotonin, dopamine, and norepinephrine metabolites have also been shown in untreated coeliacs.

Gluten can trigger depression

Rapid improvement of depressive symptoms with a gluten-free diet has been reported in some studies. Others have reported improvement of anxiety but not depression with a gluten-free diet.

There is a report of three adult patients with undiagnosed or untreated coeliac disease with depression (Corvaglia, 1999). These people did not have intestinal symptoms, but had persistent depressive symptoms. Their coeliac disease was uncovered because of their children who had been diagnosed with coeliac disease.

In all three patients, their depressive symptoms improved quickly with a gluten-free diet. They concluded that coeliac disease should be taken into consideration in the presence of behavioural and depressive disorders, particularly if they are not responsive to the usual anti-depressive therapy. Again I would go the next step and say that gluten reactions can cause this in the absence of the intestinal damage of coeliac disease.

Here are two stories of patients who have suffered depression that they have linked to eating gluten.

Jackie (35 years)

Blood tests not available
Biopsy: normal.
A depression story.

Depressed and exhausted

Jackie said: "I was plagued with postnatal depression for the first 18 months of my new baby's life. I wasn't sure if it was the demands of dealing with such a high need baby. He was never happy. He slept terribly, breastfed constantly and suffered a continuous stream of ear infections. Or was it because I was struggling to adjust to life after leaving a high-powered male-dominated profession?"

Feeling desperate

"I really couldn't think of a single nice thing to say about being a mum. So, the suggestion that my son may be gluten intolerant came as an unwelcome shock. Especially, since I was still breastfeeding him and I could hardly face giving up so many of the foods I enjoyed when I was already having such a miserable time."

Gluten-free a last resort

"We were so desperate for sleep, and this really was our last resort. So I reluctantly removed gluten from our diets. My husband and I were astonished after only one day to experience our first uninterrupted night's sleep for more than six months. Moreover, the following days we watched in wonder as a completely calm, cooperative and gentle child emerged from our son's previously aggressive and argumentative body. After a week we started to hold our breath for an ear infection, but none came, not even the following winter by which time we had been gluten-free for twelve months."

My depression lifted and disappeared

"Of course my depression lifted immediately and we put it down to the stress-free days and sleep-filled nights. I had more energy than I'd ever had in my life and positively bounced out of bed each day. My life took on a whole new dimension and I suddenly had the enthusiasm and confidence to take on all sorts of new challenges. I was finally being the sort of mum I'd always wanted to be!"

Back on gluten – back with depression

"When my son finished breastfeeding there seemed no reason for me to be gluten-free any more. So I charged back into my old eating habits, and back came the depression. I was devastated! I realized that my new-found energy, clarity and confidence were all dependent on my staying gluten-free.

"I decided to get a test for coeliac disease and was told I would have to keep eating a small amount of gluten in my diet for at least three months before taking the test. It was a long and miserable wait. I really didn't enjoy being my old, grumpy self. I was sure that the test would come back positive because the more people with coeliac disease that I spoke to, the more symptoms I realised I had."

"But the test came back negative! Even so, I know for myself that I cannot tolerate gluten in my diet. My husband notices straight away if I've cheated. And I've since realised that I even have to be careful when eating non-glutinous grains – if I overeat any gluten-free baking (that is eating other gluten-free grains) I can feel the depression right there tapping me on the shoulder."

Life without grains

"If you'd asked me five years ago to describe a diet without grain starches, I wouldn't have been able to think of a single thing to eat. But these days, I have a hard time choosing between all the delicious foods that I can eat! I am also enjoying the positive spin-offs, not least of which is the end of my weight problem that I've struggled with since I was a teenager. Now, being overweight is a thing of the past. Yes, I am finally being the sort of mum I'd always wanted to be!"

Karen (36 years)

IgG-gliadin 71   IgA-gliadin 10   tTG 6
Biopsy: not done.
Depressed and tired. Family history of gluten-sensitivity.
My story about going off gluten.

Karen was on Prozac and was unable to come off it until she went gluten-free. I had seen her children for gluten problems. Mum got tested and went gluten-free as well. She recovered, off Prozac.

Karen said: "I was feeling very, very tired and I went to the doctor and no cause was found. I had several blood tests including thyroid and iron tests. But nothing was found to explain my tiredness."

"The doctor thought I might have post-natal depression, so I was put on Prozac. I tried that for about 4–5 months. I tried coming off that and it wasn't happening very easily for me. I was having my children investigated by Doctor Rodney Ford for their problems and it was discovered that they were gluten-sensitive. Because of them, I too had a gluten blood test. It was very abnormal!. So I went gluten free when the kids did. I started the diet, and after about two months or so gluten-free, I came off the Prozac. I just weaned myself off it and I have been fine since. The tiredness that I was experiencing seems to have completely disappeared."

"I am at last well again, off gluten. It is hard to believe that such a common food could cause me so much harm. Both me and my kids are still gluten-free and we have a happy family at last. Wonderful!"

Psychiatric disorders

Schizophrenia has been associated with gluten intolerance. The diagnosis of schizophrenia describes a variety of differing individuals who belong to complex group of brain-disordered people. They often have a chronic or relapsing disease that can eventually lead to dementia. Schizophrenia is unlikely to be a single disease with a single cause.

This schizophrenic process produces a distortion of brain function. There are serious breakdowns in sensing, in feeling, in remembering, in deciding, and in acting.

Gluten-sensitivity causes milder, but similar, brain dysfunctions. This has led to the suggestion that gluten could be a trigger for setting off schizophrenia (Dohan, 1983). He states, "Considerable evidence indicates that the major cause of schizophrenia is the inborn inability to process certain digestion products of some food proteins, especially cereal grain glutens."

As with so many gluten-based hypotheses, this is regarded as controversial. However, with all of the above stories, it is inescapable that gluten harms thought and causes psychological symptoms in some people. Going gluten-free has helped huge numbers of people regain their mental health. The message is this: if you are experiencing any troubles that may be caused by brain or nerve disturbance, then get a gluten blood test.

Next, we will look at the evidence of how gut malfunctions can be attributed to nerve damage.

9. Tummy troubles

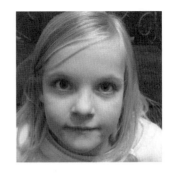

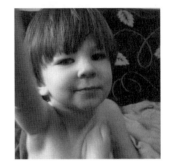

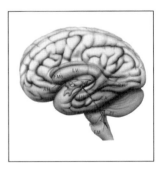

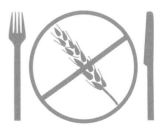

Tummy troubles

We now return to the gut. The gut is where this story began. It is the place when your food and nutrients are processed and absorbed. And finally, it is where the waste material is eliminated. It is in your gut where gluten is poorly digested. It is here where gluten can enter your blood stream and subsequently cause so much bodily upset. By now you will know all about coeliac disease. The small bowel damage is instigated by an inflammatory reaction which is spurred on by gluten in genetically susceptible people.

In my clinical work I have found that many other disorders of the gut can be caused by gluten, independent of any small bowel damage. As stated at the beginning, I believe that the explanation for these gut malfunctions is due to damage to the autonomic nervous system by gluten and the immune inflammation that it can trigger. It is also possible that the actual gluten antibody can cause damage by cross-reactivity of nerve tissue.

Gut malfunctions stem from gluten nerve damage

I have shown you that your brain carries out a myriad of regulation and control activities in the everyday function of your gut. These complex tasks happen unconsciously. You know nothing about them until they go wrong! These tasks include: peristalsis to constantly move food along your gut; oesophagus swallowing movements; stomach emptying; small bowel movement; and large bowel actions. Consequently, when these control devices are impaired by gluten, you would expect the following symptoms: gastro-oesophageal reflux and heart burn; nausea; bloating; constipation and diarrhoea. And this is indeed what you find.

Gastro-intestinal motility disorder

Coeliac patients often show gastro-intestinal motor abnormalities in clinical practice. About a half of all people with coeliac disease have now been recognised to have dyspeptic symptoms (epigastric discomfort, early satiety) which are suggestive of a gastro-intestinal motility disorder. Consistent data is now available on the presence of a disturbed motility of the oesophagus, stomach, small intestine, gallbladder, and colon of untreated coeliac patients (Tursi, 2004).

Gluten causes abnormal gut motility

Gastro-intestinal abnormalities from a malfunction of autonomic motility differ in different gastro-intestinal zones:

o   Slower oesophageal transit (slow swallowing)
o   Delayed gastric emptying (full tummy for longer)
o   Impaired gallbladder emptying (fat digestion problems)
o   Slower oro-cecal transit time (bloating)
o   Faster colonic transit (diarrhoea).

These alterations in function are the result of the complex interactions in the gastro-intestinal tract. The factors of this interweaving of function include: the reduced absorption of food nutrients (in particular, fat); neurological malfunctions; gut hormonal impairment; and small intestinal bacterial overgrowth (from the predisposing motility disorder).

The whole gut can malfunction

All of these alterations in function will disappear after a gluten-free diet is started. Again, the next insight is that all of these gut dysmotility disorders can occur in gluten-sensitivity without the additional need for small bowel histological damage.

To illustrate these gut symptoms, I have asked a number of children and parents to tell you their stories. The feature that is so impressive in these following accounts is the rapidity of symptoms with the inadvertent eating of small amounts of gluten. This means that there is some sort of amplification of the toxic effects of gluten. I am convinced that the following people experience symptoms caused by gluten in some way interfering with their autonomic nervous system function.

Gastro-oesophageal reflux

Reflux, or heartburn, occurs when the stomach contents gets pushed back up into the oesophagus. The acid in the stomach will then cause an irritation and then a burning of the skin of the oesophagus. This is very uncomfortable. It hurts. Babies scream and cry. Toddlers whine, moan and get distressed. Older children experience regurgitation of acid in their mouth. They get heartburn. They drink milk.

In my experience, both children and adults who have troublesome gastro-oesophageal reflux symptoms are frequently gluten-sensitive. Indeed, I have found that children who have severe reflux (those who require continuing treatment with acid suppressant medication past 18 months of age) nearly all turn out to be gluten-sensitive. These children have high IgG-gliadin antibody levels. When these children go onto a gluten-free diet, they settle down, they sleep well for the first time, and they begin to eat normally. They also can usually be weaned off their medications within a few weeks or months. Their parents are relieved that at last their distressing problems have been solved.

Reflux is extremely common. Anti-reflux medications are prescribed second only to pain killers. It is so common that people think that it is a "normal" symptom. From dealing with these problems every day, I have found that it is frequently precipitated by gluten.

Maddison (4 years)
IgG-Gliadin 34   IgA-gliadin 10   tTG 11
Biopsy: not done
Severe gastro-oesophageal reflux and cow's milk intolerance.

Maddison is only four years old. She has been troubled by ongoing gastro-oesophageal reflux. She tries to explain the sensation of reflux that she gets with gluten. She gets reflux when she eats gluten by error. She is gluten-sensitive.

Mum: "What happens when you get the yucky in your throat?"
Maddison said: "It hurts a little bit. I get a drink of water so it will go back down my throat. It feels a little bit yucky.
Mum: "Does it hurt?"
Maddison replies: "Yes it does. Sometimes it makes me feel a little bit angry. It makes me cry when it goes up here, because I eat too much food and it makes me sick. If I eat too much it makes it worse."

Joshua (1 year)
IgG-gliadin 91   IgA-Gliadin 72   tTG 4
Biopsy normal
Reflux, abdominal pain, cow's milk allergy and eczema

Mum said: "Josh had terrible reflux. By the time he was 10 months old the situation was getting unbearable. We had this poor little boy who was always sick and upset and as parents we were getting practically no sleep."

Help at last
"After talking to a friend we asked to be referred to a specialist, Dr Rodney Ford. Ever since that day things have constantly improved. Josh was put on the appropriate medication for his reflux and once that was under control, Josh was sent for blood tests which showed

high gluten markers. Josh also underwent a gastroscopy to look for coeliac disease – it showed that he had a normal small bowel biopsy."

A happy gluten-free boy

"After going on a gluten-free diet at 1 year old, Joshua is now a healthy and happy little boy. He hasn't been sick once in the last couple of months, his appetite is great, he sleeps for 1–2 hours during the day, waking happy. He sleeps all night in his own bed! He is happy to play on his own or with his big sister. He has such an awesome personality and a funny sense of humour. His growth has improved significantly, especially with his height. It is such a relief to have him well again. It is hard to believe that gluten was behind so many of his problems."

Constipation and soiling

When your colon is not functioning properly, you will experience constipation, soiling (encopresis), bloating, and at times diarrhoea. You also will have low immune function – the colon is a very important part of your immune system.

To empty out your colon, the large bowel muscles have to work efficiently to move the faecal contents along. You also have to be able to feel the "call to stool". That is the urge to download. I have found that the children (and adults) with constipation from gluten-sensitivity have poor sensations about wanting to defecate. They cannot feel it coming. I think that this is due to damaged nerves that control this function. Once going gluten-free, it usually takes about 3–6 months for everything to come right again.

Studies have shown that the explanation for much constipation in children is from a cow's milk protein intolerance. However, gluten is also a major contributor to this problem.

Another clue is that treatment with naloxone, a specific opioid antagonist, has been shown to benefit some children with protracted constipation (Kreek, 1983) and others with chronic irritable bowel.

The following stories are from children and a mother with troublesome symptoms from their colon. They all recovered off gluten. They had no evidence of small bowel damage.

Jasmin (5 years)

IgG-Gliadin 76   IgA-gliadin 5   tTG 5
Biopsy: not done.

Jasmin had constipation for many years and had tried all of the laxatives and high fibre diets without any improvement at all. A blood test showed a very high IgG-gliadin antibody level. Within a few months of going gluten-free she was almost better.

Eating a hot cross bun
Mum said: "At Easter time, we thought we would try her with a hot cross bun with gluten. It just blocked her up the next day! We had an absolute nightmare on our hands. That's the only full piece of bread or gluten product she has had since Christmas time, four months ago."

"She had terrible constipation, but after going gluten-free she became normal again. Since going gluten-free she has changed her focus on life. Her focus is no longer on doing poos. Her focus used to be on trying to do poos and she would complain about her sore bottom all the time."

"Now, going to the toilet is not an issue! She will go away to the toilet and there is no problem at all. What a relief! Before, her whole life used to revolve around the toilet, but now she is just great. Perhaps the best thing of all is that she is just loving school."

James (8 years)

IgG-gliadin 84   IgA-gliadin 8   tTG 5
Biopsy: not done.
Soiling with bowel motions, abdominal pain.

Soiling for six months
Mum said: "For about six months, James was embarrassed because he had lost control of his bowel motions. He was soiling and was beginning to smell. He is a very shy boy anyway and this was a difficulty added to him at school."

"On a suggestion from his grandmother he went gluten-free and almost immediately his tummy pains disappeared and he had less soiling. He had a blood test that showed he had a very high gluten antibody and was then put on a strict gluten-free diet."

Better within days off gluten
"Amazingly, within a few days he had stopped soiling. His tummy pains disappeared. Now, he seems extremely sensitive to gluten. When he takes a small amount of gluten by accident, within about five minutes he has to rush off to the toilet because he gets diarrhoea."

Dry at night too
"Also, I am very pleased because he is now dry at night. This is the first time ever. Perhaps his gluten-free diet is helping with his bladder control. The whole family has gone gluten-free now and they feel much better. His dad had tummy cramps and they have gone."

Lachlan (4 years)

IgG-gliadin 6   IgA-gliadin 5   tTG 5
Biopsy: not done.

Lachlan is gluten-sensitive. He was being looked after by the baby-sitter who mistakenly gave him a gluten biscuit! He had been strictly gluten-free. He developed severe abdominal pain and was hospitalised. This is a good illustration about the devastating effects that gluten can cause.

He ate some gluten
Mum said: "Our baby-sitter had two lots of food out for the night: hers, with wheat based products; and food for the children which was gluten-free. My children obviously talked her into giving them some gluten biscuits (or they just took them). The next day, at 4 pm, his sore tummy came on suddenly. That night, I couldn't touch Lachlan even gently. He was in so much pain. He was groaning and moaning."

Something serious
"Lachlan doesn't complain about stuff, it takes a lot to bring him down. So I took him to the After Hours medical service at 4.30 pm. He was still groaning and groaning, but worse. He was pointing to his tummy, he said it was very sore. He couldn't go to the toilet to do a poo although he wanted to. He fell asleep."

"About an hour later we got through to the doctor who wasn't sure if it was constipation, or appendicitis, or a twisted bowel or a twisted testicle. He thought it was something serious. We couldn't wake Lachlan up – but if you touched him, he winced with pain."

Going to hospital with constipation!
"So, we were sent off to the hospital! While we were waiting, he slept for quite some time. At last, hours later, he woke up. The doctors then were preparing him for an emergency operation to find

out what was wrong. They asked him if he needed to go to the toilet – they wanted to take a sample. So he did, and we took a sample, and the sample came back okay. After that he perked up and was fine! They sent him home with some medication to make him go to the toilet."

I felt stupid saying that this was a reaction to gluten
"I had spent six hours in the hospital that night. I felt that I should have said something about gluten. I thought about it. Do I say it or do I not. I felt so stupid. The doctors said that it was "Just constipation!" I should have said about the gluten but I didn't think that they would have believed me."

Caitlin (6 years)

IgG-gliadin 87   IgA-gliadin 7   tTG 3
Biopsy: not done.

Caitlin had been struggling with constipation all of her life. Her mother said this about Caitlin gaining sensation in her bowel soon after going gluten-free.

Mum said: "After being gluten-free, Caitlin who has not been bowel or urine continent her whole life – well she has gained sensation to her bowel motions! And she also goes to the toilet to do wees!"

Better in just weeks
"It only took about two weeks of going gluten-free before she started feeling her poos for the first time. It was miraculous!"

"If she now takes gluten by mistake she really knows about it. Within 15–20 minutes she has horrendous stomach cramps. Within an hour or so she has diarrhoea which she has no control over. She also gets severe headaches. She is the best that she has ever been now that she is gluten-free."

Esther (8 years)

IgG-gliadin 37   IgA-gliadin 55   tTG 11
Endomysial antibodies negative.
Biopsy: not done.

Esther always had bowel troubles. She had constipation, abdominal pain, encopresis, and a poor appetite. Going gluten-free has changed her life.

Mum says: "We found out that Esther was gluten intolerant at Christmas time. We had taken her off gluten. Previously, Esther had a lot of trouble with her bowels, a lot of trouble passing her motions. Off gluten, we found that it has taken about 3 or 4 months and now we don't have any problems. She doesn't have any messes on her underwear. That used to happen a lot, but now she can actually pass the motion. She can feel it."

"I found that she has a lot more energy which is really good. And her skin is coming right. Like her skin on her body even on her chest and back was very dry and scaly. That has come right. Her arms seem to be taking a bit longer to heal."

"Not long ago she had some gluten by mistake – she ate a gluten saveloy. Within about an hour she got so sore in her tummy, she felt like being sick, but she didn't spew up."

Esther said: "Gluten is not very good for me. I now have a happy tummy. Yeah!"

In summary, in my experience, I have seen hundreds of children with chronic, intractable constipation that has completely got better when they go onto a gluten-free diet. Nearly all of these children have high IgG-gliadin antibodies. They take up to six months to completely improve.

Diarrhoea and abdominal pain

Diarrhoea refers to having loose bowel motions, also called loose stools. "Runny poos" is a common term used by children and parents. Sometimes there can be a sense of urgency and loss of control can occur. It is a very common symptom and has many possible causes.

Loose bowels motions, as a symptom of coeliac disease, are mostly due to the poor absorption of food nutrients from the gut. All of this undigested food in the large bowel causes havoc. It gets fermented by the bacteria in the colon, creating rectal gas and more fluid. The tummy gets distended and the bowel motions can be explosive.

However, when the small bowel is not damaged, nevertheless, diarrhoea can still occur. This can be due to the irritation of the nerve networks of the intestine that will then try to quickly expel the unwanted foods. This is the explanation for tiny amounts of gluten causing large amounts of diarrhoea and abdominal pain.

Abdominal pain that is generated within the gut is derived from spasm of intestinal muscles; or from distention and stretching of the bowel wall; or from inflammation of the surrounding tissues, nerves and glands. Stimulation of the autonomic nervous system can also cause a gut ache. Spasms of the muscles and distention by too much gas will give you a colicky pain – these are sharp intermittent pains that often come in waves. When you get these pains it makes you want to double up.

Pains generated from the inflammation of tissues are more constant and there is a tendency for you to remain still. Pain in the oesophagus is sometimes called heart burn. In children, this causes them to squirm, cry or arch their body backwards. Gluten has been implicated as a factor in all of these types of pains. Here are some more stories from a number of people who have suffered from diarrhoea and abdominal pains from eating small amounts of gluten.

Tayla (7 years)

IgG-gliadin 86   IgA-gliadin 10   tTG 7
Endomysial antibodies negative.
Biopsy: not done.

Tayla had been gluten-free for about a year. She used to have tummy pains and get tired and unwell. Blood tests showed that she was gluten-sensitive and she recovered within a few weeks when she went gluten-free. It was now time to test out if she was okay with a small amount of gluten.

Urgent diarrhoea within 30 minutes
Tayla said: "I went to a restaurant and mum said I could try a little bit of that hot-dog and a chicken nugget. We knew that there was gluten in it. I was playing with the other children when I suddenly had a sore tummy. Mum says that it all happened in about half an hour. The pain was in the middle of my tummy, near my tummy button."

"I went to the toilet and had lots and lots of runny poos. It was very smelly. And my tummy was tight. There was no swelling, but it felt rock hard. The next day I was okay."

Mum said: "She came running to me and said, "I really need to go to the toilet – I need to go!" It was urgent. Then she said, "I need your help, mum, quickly". I went with her to the toilet and she had a really sore tummy and diarrhoea. "Since then she has stayed gluten free!"

Joanne (36 years)

IgG-gliadin 19   IgA-gliadin 13   tTG 25
Bloods taken after being gluten-free for five years.
Biopsy: coeliac disease.

My last gluten mistake – a terrible tummy
"I have been gluten-free for about five years now. I have not had many accidents."

Eating out ends in terrible pain
"Last month I had lunch out with a friend. By the time I was heading home, it would be probably an hour or so later, I started getting my pains. I get a bad pain on the right side of my tummy. I got progressively worse and by the time I got home I had terrible pains and also diarrhoea."

"I rang the restaurant where we had lunch. I knew straight away that they had put an extra salad out. It was a different salad with some wheat in it. I had eaten about a spoonful. I was subsequently in and out of bed for two days. I then had pains and diarrhoea for about three days. And then I was tired for about another ten days after that. This was a "gluten-free restaurant", apparently. They are really so good normally. It was such a surprise to get so unwell."

I am very sensitive
"Initially, I was very sensitive when I went gluten-free. I would only have to eat a tiny bit of gluten and I would have pains. It seems that I am still very sensitive!"

"I had an endoscopy. My biopsy was abnormal – I had no villi. I definitely have coeliac disease. Gluten really upsets me really, really quickly. I had such low energy for a couple of weeks after that last gluten attack."

Niquaila (3 years)

IgG-Gliadin 28   IgA-gliadin 7   tTG 5
Biopsy: not done.

She stole a bread roll

Mum said: "We were at a wedding and she ate a bread roll! She was running around and playing with the other children. She must have decided that she was far too busy to eat her special food. She saw a bread roll. Her eyes lit up. She thought that would be great."

"Her mother (me!!) let her have it. I thought that it was better to have something in her tummy than nothing. Oh dear! What a lesson it was to me."

Three days of diarrhoea

"For three days she had severe diarrhoea and it took another three days to clear up and get her tummy back to normal again. This shows me that she has now become more sensitive to gluten, having gone off gluten for about six months now. Her mood over those few days was worse, but it could have gone hand in hand with the late night as well from the wedding. It was a 10 pm night."

Sore tummy too

"She complained of a sore tummy for days. It was a really good learning experience for her because she had eaten no other gluten around it. It was clearly the bread roll that did it. Even her preschool teacher said to me: "Are you aware that your daughter has got really bad diarrhoea". Yes I did! I told her that she had eaten some gluten and that it will be about two more days – then she will be fine."

"It is surprising how quickly these symptoms can come on with seemingly disproportionate amounts of gluten eaten. Why did such a small amount cause her so much upset?"

Abdominal migraine

The term abdominal migraine has been used to describe recurrent abdominal pain with no other apparent cause. A tummy headache. It got this name because the pain could be severe and associated with nausea. Sometimes a headache would arise as well.

In the headache literature, abdominal migraine is defined as one of the variants of migraine headache. It is also known by other terms including "periodic syndrome." This variant is said to be seen most typically in children. People who have abdominal migraine usually have a family history of headache migraine. They often go on to develop typical migraine later in their life.

The attacks of abdominal migraine are characterised by periodic bouts of abdominal pain which usually last for a few hours. In addition to the abdominal pain, these sufferers may have other symptoms such as nausea and vomiting, flushing or pallor.

Traditional tests have failed to reveal a cause for this pain. However, occasionally there are EEG findings that are suggestive of epilepsy – but this is rarely related to any convulsions. The usual medical practice is to put such children on long-term medications that are used for treating migraine. These medications do lessen these attacks in most children. Indeed, that is why these abdominal attacks are called abdominal migraine! They appear to be generated within the tummy brain – probably neurological activity triggered by gluten.

My hypothesis is that the seat of gluten-sensitivity is in the autonomic nervous system. This is exactly where these abdominal migraines are likely to originate. In my experience, nearly all of these children are gluten-sensitive. They have high IgG-gliadin antibodies and immediately get completely better on a gluten-free diet.

10. Got it! Grains and your brain

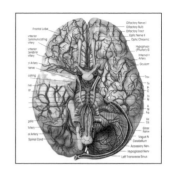

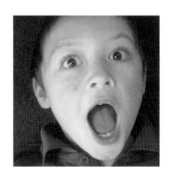

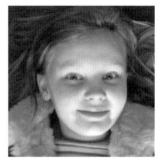

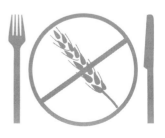

10. Got it!

Grains and your brains

By now you will have read about the common brain and gut reactions that I, and many others, believe are frequently sparked off by eating gluten. Of course, not all such symptoms can be blamed on gluten – but there is a strong case that at least one in ten people are so affected.

I have come to this conclusion through my clinical work in food allergy. I have looked after thousands of children and their parents by understanding how foods have been making them sick and tired. Gluten has become the number one problem. Gluten is causing widespread damage to millions of people.

The shocking truth about gluten

The shocking truth for me is that this terrible scourge of gluten is being ignored by most medical practitioners. Even worse, the blood test that can diagnose it is being abandoned by many laboratories. The problem is also being made worse by food manufacturers who are adding gluten to so many processed foods. Gluten foods have steadily become a big part of the staple diet. The other fearsome news is that it can so seriously affect your brain and nerves.

Have you got it?

By now you will have got the message that gluten can damage your brain. So you will have been asking yourself "Have I got it?" You will want to know the answer to the question, "How can I get tested?" You will want to know if you should go gluten-free, and how long would it be before you get better.

The critics

There is no lack of critics of this gluten story. The medical profession is rightly very conservative and demands a high standard of proof before changing guidelines. But how much proof is necessary?

However, there is an entrenched position on coeliac disease. The currently held "medical" belief is that coeliac disease is only a gut disease and that the only role for a gluten-free diet is for the treatment of a person with the biopsy-proven histological damage of coeliac disease. I disagree. This book has been written to reveal the much wider view on gluten-sensitivity.

The criticisms

It is easy to be critical. It is comfortable to oppose changing ideas. I need to be courageous in putting forward a whole new way of thinking about gluten. The criticisms that I regularly get are these.

a) The benefits that your patients get are subjective.
Yes, their results are subjective. In the opinion of the patient, or parent or child, they feel better and are grateful that all of their symptoms have disappeared. What clinches it for me is that these families are willing to persevere on an extremely strict gluten-free diet for years. They find that even small infringements will cause a relapse.

b) The benefits are due to my observation bias.
Yes, I am biased. I am enthusiastic. I am an encourager. However, I attempt to be as unbiased in my clinical assessment as I can be. This bias would be an important factor if my results had been borderline. However, I have been overwhelmed by the numbers of children and adults who have made amazing recoveries on a gluten-free diet. Previously, they had experienced ill health for years or even decades. Nothing else had helped them.

c) The benefits are due to a healthier diet.

Yes, this is true. A healthier diet will contribute to better health. I emphasize to my patients the need to ensure that iron deficiency and other mineral/vitamin deficits are restored. Iron repletion makes a huge difference. However, gluten-sensitivity is usually the cause of the low iron. And again, these families find that even small traces of gluten will cause a setback. This is despite going onto a more healthy diet.

d) The benefits are due to a more strict control of the children.

Yes, in other studies, more attention to parenting and more positive time spent with children will show benefits in behaviour. This does certainly occur when they spend more time preparing food and making sure that their children are eating well. However, yet again the parents find that the reintroduction of gluten is associated with a relapse. Even tiny amounts.

e) We require a double-blind randomised control trial.

Yes, randomised control challenges are a very good way to get objective results. These types of study are the mainstay of much medical research – especially drug trials. Briefly, to do such a study the patients would be randomly split into two groups. One group gets gluten-free foods. The other group gets gluten-containing foods. Which group you are in is kept a secret from you and the study observers until the end of the trial. In my opinion, my observations are so strong that I feel it is not ethical to knowingly deprive someone of the very real benefits of a gluten-free diet. Also the difficulties of a double-blind diet of gluten-free would be an almost impossible study to set up. Capsules of gluten would need to be given. Everyone would get so ill. Frankly, I do not think that it is worth that effort when the results of a gluten-free diet are so plainly obvious.

f) They would have got better anyway.
Yes, some of these people might have got better anyway. However, most come to see me following months, years or even decades of illness and suffering. After a full medical assessment and blood tests, if they seem to be gluten-sensitive, I commence them on a three-month gluten-free diet. The astonishing fact is that nearly all such people get better within weeks (the younger the person, the more quickly they improve). If this response happened occasionally, then it might be coincidence. But I see these "cures" time and time again. I attribute their miraculous improvement to the gluten-free diet. And again, if they infringe, then they relapse.

g) Gluten-free is too much of an imposition on these families.
No! I disagree. I too used to think that the gluten-free diet was a major burden. But it is not. Only a few children jack up about it. The adults are relieved to at last be on a program that gives them a new life. Nowadays, there are so many good gluten-free products which are widely available. The first few weeks are the most difficult. Then it becomes easy. In my experience, people usually eat more healthily on a gluten-free diet. Also, to overcome the initial difficulties, we have written a starter book that explains the diet in a straightforward manner (Going gluten-free: how to get started). A gluten-free diet is now easy. Carrying it on for years and years is where it can be more challenging. There are also some social drawbacks – but these are nothing compared with the benefits that are experienced.

h) Any diet works.
I disagree. Many of my patients have been on all sorts of diets without the relief that they have been searching for. Once a certain diagnosis of gluten-sensitivity has been made, then they find it much easier to follow the new food restriction. Better at last!

i) The IgG-gliadin is a nonspecific test and has little to do with gluten-sensitivity.

I disagree. I have been investigating this test for over five years. Almost invariably I find that if someone has symptoms, and they have a high IgG-gliadin antibody level, then they will respond favourably to a gluten-free diet. On the other hand, if they have a normal IgG-gliadin, they usually do not respond. However, this is not always the case. Unfortunately, many laboratories are now discontinuing the IgG-gliadin test as it is not diagnostic of coeliac disease. However, the widespread community recognition of gluten-sensitivity will turn this tide.

j) A high IgG-gliadin just reflects increased gut permeability.

I don't think so. It is my belief that the high IgG-gliadin is because of the disordered permeability. However, the important information that I am trying to get through is that this high IgG-gliadin antibody level is a very useful blood test to find a huge group of patients who respond positively to a gluten-free diet. In the diseases where the gut is inflamed and leaky, then gluten-sensitivity may play an important role in the symptoms. Gluten reactions may make the underlying illness a lot worse. Also, the gluten antibody itself maybe harmful to nerve networks.

k) This brain story is unjustified speculation.

I disagree. I believe that I have argued my case well. There is strong evidence from a huge accumulation of information: from patient symptoms; from neurological clinics; from brain scan studies; from postmortems; from nerve cell histology; from brain cell physiology; and from the amazing responses of following a gluten-free diet. Your brain and nerve tissues are responsible for the regulation of your body. When they go wrong, you can develop a myriad of symptoms such as are experienced in gluten-sensitivity.

l) A crack pot idea.

I disagree. This is the easiest criticism to make. An attempt to discredit the idea and the person behind it. This always happens with every new idea. The conservatives do not like the changes that any new thinking brings. New thoughts might make the old ways irrelevant. They might have to make changes themselves. What they are doing currently might then be regarded as wrong. There are always obstacles put in the path of progress.

More answers to your questions

You probably have a lot more questions. Here are answers to some of the most common questions that I am asked. More detail is given in my other books. If you have a question, please ask it.

Ask your gluten questions

How can you tell if you are being damaged by gluten?

Simply, if you (or your child) have any of the ongoing symptoms listed in the first chapter, then you should organise to get your blood tests. Because gluten-sensitivity causes such a wide range of symptoms, it cannot be accurately diagnosed by just listening.

Who should get a blood test?

I believe that everyone who suffers from any chronic ill health should get a test for IgG-gliadin antibodies. In my experience, you cannot tell unless you test. The problem is that so many people who have poor health and low energy think that they are "normal". I encourage people who want to experience more energy and more vitality to also get their blood tested. Many are positive to gluten!

Can I go gluten-free without a blood test?

No! You must get a blood test. There are many people with coeliac disease who have few or even no symptoms. Before going gluten-free you want to know whether or not you have coeliac disease. If you do, then you will need to be on a strict gluten-free diet for life – no exceptions. The blood test is to help you with the future and for an accurate diagnosis.

Always get a blood test first

What do antibody blood tests show?

This is covered in Chapter 2. Briefly, the antibody tests look for two distinctly different reactions. The gluten antibodies (especially, IgG-gliadin) indicate the body's immunologic reaction to gluten that you eat in your diet. If you have never had gluten, then you cannot be reactive to gluten.

IgG-gliadin test is essential

The tissue antibodies (tissue transglutaminase and endomesial antibodies) give evidence about the tissue damage in the small bowel. If these tissue markers are high, then it is likely that the person has coeliac disease (also called gluten-sensitive enteropathy). People with coeliac disease usually also have high levels of gluten antibodies.

What blood tests should I get?

The most important point of getting blood tests is to confirm or deny coeliac disease. This is crucial. Do not go on a gluten-free diet without first having the blood tests. The other reason for blood tests is to confirm gluten-sensitivity. Checking your iron levels and immune function is important too. To achieve this, you need all of the tests that are detailed in Chapter 1.

Are blood tests infallible?

No! Blood tests are very good, but not one hundred percent reliable. If all of your blood tests are normal, you still could be gluten-sensitive. Often, a whole family will decide to go gluten-free. They may all feel a benefit from the diet, although some members might have normal coeliac and gluten blood tests.

Gluten-free suits lots of people

Can I have a blood test if I am already gluten-free?

Yes. Probably. It depends how long you have been on the diet, how strictly, and what answer you are seeking. Most people in this situation want to know if they have coeliac disease. It takes over a year for very abnormal blood tests to go down to near normal levels. For some, their blood tests do not normalize for two or three years. Therefore, blood tests are of some value within the first year of going gluten-free. Doing HLA gene testing can also contribute to the diagnostic picture.

How do I read my own blood tests?

Currently, the focus on blood tests that look at gluten issues is on making the diagnosis of coeliac disease. Unfortunately, the IgG-gliadin tests are not very useful in making such a diagnosis (the tissue antibodies, such as tTG, are much more specific). The upshot of this is that the IgG-gliadin test results are usually disregarded. The medical practitioners have been told that an isolated high IgG-gliadin test is a "false positive". They are told that it does not mean anything. Moreover, the diagnosis of gluten-sensitivity is not yet being made by mainstream medicine. This is because there has not been enough written about it in the traditional medical literature.

Check out the lab

Even worse, is that many laboratories are now refusing to do this test because of cost-cutting policies. This is because the IgG-gliadin is said not to contribute to the diagnosis of coeliac disease (I disagree!). So at present getting your blood tests can be difficult.

How common is being gluten-sensitive?

I believe that at least one in ten people are adversely affected by gluten. I have calculated this from the patients that get referred to my clinic. For every one child I see with coeliac disease, there are ten others who I diagnose with gluten-sensitivity. Coeliac disease has been shown to occur in about one in a hundred people. Gluten-sensitivity is ten times more common.

One in ten are gluten-sensitive

Is the brain damage permanent?

It could be. This cannot be answered in full yet. It is my observation that the younger the person who is put on a gluten-free diet, the better response they experience, and the more quickly they recover. This is to be expected because once brain and nerve inflammation becomes entrenched, then the likelihood of a full recovery becomes more remote. Most of the brain recovery data in the literature is based on adult studies. I would expect a much more optimistic view once the childhood gluten-sensitive children are discovered and treated with a gluten-free diet.

What if I make a mistake?

Nothing much! There is no danger of long-term damage. You (or your child) might get a few symptoms and feel unwell for a bit. But it soon passes. However, it is important that gluten infringements do not creep up and become common. This is especially important with those with a coeliac disease diagnosis.

Who in the family should get a gluten blood test?

Gluten-Sensitivity runs in the family. I recommend that everyone in a family who has coeliac disease or gluten-sensitivity should get a blood test. Also, by doing gluten blood tests on everyone in my clinic, I discover a parent with coeliac disease every week or so. I repeat – "If you don't have a blood test, then you will never know."

Gluten-sensitivity runs in families

What is a wheat-free diet?

A wheat-free diet is different to a gluten-free diet. A wheat-free diet is not gluten-free. But it is sometimes recommended if there is a specific allergy to wheat. I rarely see this problem. It is more common in babies with eczema. If you have a positive blood test to gluten, then you need a gluten-free diet.

167

Can gluten-sensitivity emerge at any age?

Coeliac disease and gluten-sensitivity are conditions that can be seen as "a work in progress". No one is born with coeliac disease or with gluten-sensitivity. But it develops as your immune system matures and causes an antibody reaction to gluten in your diet. If you remain gluten-free lifelong then you cannot develop these conditions.

Symptoms can develop at any age

Gluten-sensitivity can very often occur in the first couple of years of life. Coeliac disease often presents at that time too. However, the symptoms can be quite subtle and it can be discovered at any age at all. In my experience, I am diagnosing people as young as nine months and as old as 70 years. It may be that when the bowel is damaged by infection, that it is more open to gluten passing through the gut wall which can cause an immune reaction. This may be an explanation for the later onset of some gluten-sensitivity problems.

How does gluten affect my gut?

Briefly, if you have the coeliac gene, then gluten can be directly toxic to your gut. If you have the gluten-sensitive picture, then it is my belief that gluten harms the nerves that control your gut – this causes your gut's functions to break down and bring about all of your symptoms. The only way to treat this is to go on a strict gluten-free diet!

Most symptoms are from nerve dysfunction

What about wheat products in shampoos and cosmetics?

Usually, gluten in these products does not matter much. However, some people are very sensitive and they get itchy skin with gluten containing cosmetics and shampoos. Lipsticks are more of a problem because the gluten can be ingested (by you or your partner!).

How do I start to go gluten-free?

I have now helped thousands of people to go gluten-free. I began to feel guilty about this – and so I too went on a gluten-free diet. It was not as difficult as I was expecting it to be. I learned a lot from this experience, and with my wife, Chris, we wrote about our experiences in our book "Going gluten-free: how to get started." The first day we both felt overwhelmed as our brains suddenly had to adjust to new patterns of shopping, cooking and eating.

Take your time

However, within a few days we were already getting into the swing of it. Our most important bit of advice is not to hurry it. You do not have to be perfect on the first day. You will make lots and lots of mistakes – but that does not matter. As the days go by, you will become more and more expert. We are all human and will get tripped up. It is much easier than you might think.

How strict does my gluten-free diet have to be?

It depends upon why you are on a gluten-free diet. If you have coeliac disease – then you need a very strict gluten-free diet, lifelong. But if you are gluten-sensitive (that means you have no gut damage) then you perhaps can eat gluten to tolerance. But see below.

How long do I have to be gluten-free?

If you have coeliac disease, then you need to commit to a strict gluten-free diet lifelong. That is forever. The long term follow up information shows that you need to remain gluten-free to stay in great health. That is even if gluten does not seem to cause you any symptoms. Gluten-sensitivity, without gut damage, and without evidence of the coeliac gene, is a different story.

Stay gluten free for a long time

No one knows the answer. It is my experience to date that those who are affected do not develop tolerance. Also, with so much evidence that gluten can cause nerve and brain damage, I think that it would be prudent to stay gluten-free for a very long time.

Should everyone have a small bowel biopsy?

No. In my opinion, not everyone needs to have a small bowel biopsy. However, it is an extremely important investigation. It should not be rejected lightly.

I advise a small bowel biopsy for all children and adults who have elevated tTG or EMA antibodies. Also in those who have substantially elevated IgA-gliadin levels or very high IgG-antigliadin levels. With the advent of coeliac "gene" testing by HLA type, I use this result to guide me on who is most likely to benefit from a small bowel biopsy.

However, endoscopy is not only about the small bowel. It also gives the opportunity to look for inflammation in the oesophagus and stomach. Many of these gluten-sensitive children present with symptoms of gastro-oesophageal reflux or gastritis.

Can you tell me about food additives and gluten?

This is a very common question, and perhaps the most complicated. The 1400 range of food additives are the "thickeners". The problem is that these are made from starch and thus may contain gluten.

Thickeners are additives used in food manufacturing that thicken and give a smooth uniform texture to a food. For instance, thickeners are often added to sauces, mayonnaises, pie fillings, dairy desserts, custards, yoghurts, soups – lots and lots of processed foods contain thickeners.

Additive numbers 1400–1450 are called thickeners. They are made from "starch". Therefore, they may be made from wheat starch. If they are wheat-based, then they will contain very small levels of gluten. And so these thickeners are not gluten free.

But, and here is the confusion, if these thickeners are derived from other starches such as maize, potato, tapioca or rice, then they are gluten-free. So sometimes these thickeners are gluten-free.

This means that you do have to read the food label carefully. Food labelling laws now require wheat-derived thickeners to be declared in the ingredients listing. Another confusion is that thickeners are sometimes called "modified starch" or "dextrins". The most important advice is this: if the source of the thickener comes from wheat (or another gluten-containing grain), then it should be avoided on the gluten free diet.

The final confusion is this: all thickeners with numbers outside the 1400–1450 range are gluten-free. These new thickeners also include 181 (tannin), 400–418, (vegetable gums), 440 (pectin), and 461–466 (celluloses). These are gluten free!

The gluten-sensitive patients

The storytellers

I thank the children and their parents who so willingly wrote down their experiences about being gluten-sensitive. They told their story to help you. Hearing the problem in their own words is helpful and refreshing.

The blood test information of these people who told their stories has been put together so that you can see the distribution of their blood tests. They did not all have blood tests. Of the 29 people, blood tests were available for 25, of whom some were already on a gluten-free diet.

Most had blood tests for IgG-gliadin and tTG (or EMA). Many had a small bowel biopsy. Two had coeliac disease. They all made a clinical response to a gluten-free diet. Finally, they had agreed to tell their story.

The blood tests

The focus of this analysis is to present the *clinical* value of the IgG-gliadin test. All IgG-gliadin, IgA-gliadin and tTG antibody measurements were performed using the assay ELISA kit from INOVA Diagnostics, San Diego, CA, USA.

The blood tests of all 25 people who had these measurements are given. I repeat, only two had a definite diagnosis of coeliac disease.

Blood tests are essential for diagnosis

---

tTG results

Results of the tTG tests are reported first, because this is the most specific and accurate test for coeliac disease.

The tTG levels for all 25 children and adults are shown in *Figure 1*. The tTG levels give the information as expected, with the two coeliacs tested having elevated levels. Both had an abnormal biopsy.

For the gluten-sensitive people, their tTG measurements were at normal levels (less than 20 units). This demonstrates the value of the tTG test which is highly reliable at identifying tissue damage. But it is not useful in the diagnosis of gluten-sensitivity. These gluten-sensitive storytellers did not have coeliac disease.

Figure 1. **tTG by age for all 25 people**

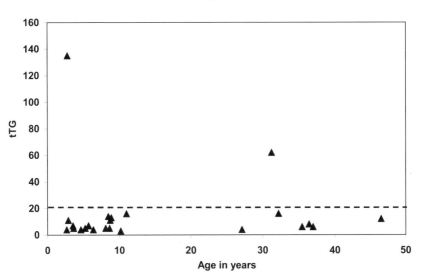

IgG-gliadin results

Figure 2 shows the IgG-gliadin blood results of this group of 25 storytellers. Nearly all had levels above 20 units (the stated "normal limit"). However, in children I find the level of 10 units to be the clinical cutoff (using INOVA Diagnostics assay kits).

There was a wide range of IgG-gliadin levels. There were two people with "normal" levels. They had already been on a gluten-free diet for some time.

The child and adult ranges of IgG-gliadin are similar. Also, the coeliac disease children have the same range of IgG-gliadin as the gluten-sensitive children. This data demonstrates the immense clinical value of the IgG-gliadin test in making the diagnosis of gluten-sensitivity.

Figure 2. IgG-gliadin by age for all 25 people

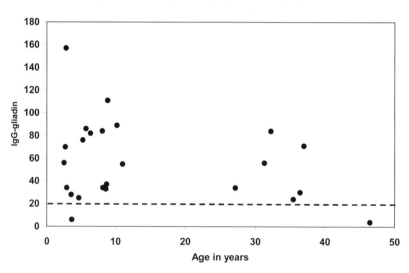

IgA-gliadin results

IgA-gliadin levels for these 25 subjects are shown in *Figure 3*.

The stated "normal" level with this test system was less than 15 units. The IgA-gliadin test did not contribute as much to the diagnosis. However, it gives added suspicion that there could be a significant reaction to gluten. It is a useful adjunct to the other tests. Almost always, high levels are associated with high levels of IgG-gliadin.

A high IgA-gliadin level is an indication for endoscopy.

These gliadin antibodies levels slowly go down once a gluten-free diet has started. They reach normal levels after a year or so. These antibodies indicate an immune reaction to gluten.

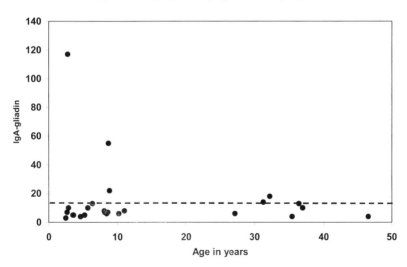

Figure 3.   IgA-gliadin by age for all 25 people

Fantastic responses to gluten-free diets

When these children were initially taken off gluten, this is what their parents said. It is truly amazing that these changes were seen so quickly on a gluten-free diet.

The phrases that follow are the verbatim comments from these people experiencing changes on a gluten-free diet:

> Terrible migraines almost gone.
> Better! School back to normal, tummy pains gone.
> Happy again.
> Huge difference. Much more energy, incredible, amazing.
> Bowels now normal.
> Huge change, more energy, concentration better.
> Personality has come back, less sore tummies.
> He is a lot better. Lost his aches and pains.
> Yes! More energy, appetite improved.
> Much better. Very sensitive to gluten.
> Fantastic difference, happy, giggling.
> Behaviour so much better.
> Big difference, more energy, bright and attentive.
> More energy, no heartburn and headaches gone.
> A different person, great behaviour, more energy.
> Doing well at school.
> Been really good, heaps better, moods better.
> Much better but still needs omeprazole.
> Behaviour generally a lot better.
> Much better with tummy pains gone and normal bowels.
> More energy.
> Absolutely fantastic off gluten after five days.
> Dramatic changes. More energy. Less irritable.

Last words

The world is full of it! The world is full of people who are reacting badly to the gluten in their diet. The shocking truth about gluten is that this phenomenon has been going on almost completely unrecognised.

Many of the ideas behind this book came from discussions with my colleague Professor Ron Harper, who wrote the foreword to this book. He and I were seeing people suffering from the same symptoms. I saw these people from the gastroenterology and food allergy angle. He was looking at these same problems from his brain physiology know-how.

Then the penny dropped! The gut troubles, and nearly all of the other symptoms due to gluten, could be caused by disordered brain and nerve network control. That was an exciting day! We rushed off to see what had been published on this topic.

This book is the result of this pivotal insight and the subsequent investigation. This book is all about how gluten-grains can damage your brain. We have reviewed the world medical literature on how gluten is associated with a vast number of brain diseases and symptoms.

Our diets are full of it – full of gluten! So many people are full of sickness through eating gluten. The underlying hypothesis is that all of this illness is caused by gluten (and perhaps gluten antibodies) damaging the brain and nerve tissues. We believe that we have presented our case well. There is a vast amount of circumstantial evidence pointing to the nervous system as the prime site of gluten damage. So, if you are sick and tired – then go and get a blood test. One in ten people are affected by gluten.

One of the shocking truths about gluten-sensitivity is the scale of the problem. It is hard to believe that one in ten people suffer from gluten-sensitivity. But that is what the figures show. We are not alone in making such an estimate. Others would put this figure even higher.

We are excited that we have discovered the mechanism to explain the very wide spectrum of gluten illness. This is an epidemic. We are full of the desire to pass this information onto others. We are full of expectation that this new found knowledge will help so many people.

However, as in all such moves forward, we expect a sizable opposition. The diagnosis of gluten-sensitivity is not yet sanctioned by the wider medical community. It will take many years before this gluten knowledge becomes incorporated into mainstream diagnoses. The next step is to encourage other research groups to carefully examine this hypothesis of a brain-grain connection. At this stage we have generated more questions than answers.

Personally, after managing thousands of patients with gluten-sensitivity, I am utterly convinced that gluten is a leading cause of behaviour, mood and energy problems. My hope is that this book will in some way make a difference to you, the reader.

You could be the one

Perhaps the most important lesson to learn is to always consider the possibility of gluten-sensitivity in anyone who has chronic ill health or neurological problems. Check out your gluten blood tests. Yes, you could be the one!

Natalie's brown bread

This is our favourite bread – it works every time

Place into a bowl the following:
> 2 cups of warm water *or* milk
> 1 Tablespoon brown sugar
> 1 ¼ teaspoon yeast (GF)
> 1 egg
> 3 Tablespoons of oil
> Approx 500gms GF bread mix (e.g. Healtheries)
>   *or* half bread mix and half baking mix
> 1 heaped Tablespoon coarse *maize* cornmeal
> 1 heaped Tablespoon fine *maize* cornmeal *or* rice flour
> 1 heaped Tablespoon ground linseed
> 1 heaped Tablespoon sunflower seeds
> 1 heaped Tablespoon pumpkin seeds [optional]
> 1 teaspoon guar gum.

Mix ingredients gently together.
Scrape the firmish mixture into your bread maker 'bucket' and cook on the rapid programme with dark crust (some other bread-makers might use the 'basic' programme for best results).

If your bread sinks in centre it may be too moist at the start. You can also use the light crust and large loaf setting for Panasonic bread makers.

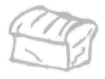

Variations on Natalie's brown bread recipe

This has been our most popular bread – people tell us that it was the breakthrough that they were looking for.

A mum who has just started her gluten-free diet sent us this message:

"I have made this recipe everyday for the last month, and it never fails. My four kids love the bread, and have it as sandwiches in their lunchboxes every day. Their favourite is ham and cheese.

This loaf is slightly sweet but you can adjust the amount of sugar according to taste.

If you make a wetter mixture, then the loaf turns out lighter
If the mixture is drier, then the loaf is dense.

I sometimes substitute the Tablespoon of ground linseed and the Tablespoon of sunflower seeds for 2 Tablespoons of LSA meal (ground Linseed, ground Sunflower seeds and blanched Almonds) which is readily available in supermarkets.

This is such a successful bread.

The kids forget that they are eating gluten-free!"

Enjoy!

References

Apley, John. Paediatrics.
Book. 1979. 2nd ed. Pub. Bailliere Tindall. UK

Blaxill Mark F.
What's Going On? The Question of Time Trends in Autism. 537
Public Health Reports Volume 119. November–December 2004

Bodé S, Gudmand-Hoyer E.
Symptoms and haematological features in consecutive adult
coeliac patients.
Scand J Gastroenterol 1996; 3: 54-60.

Bozzola M, Giovenale D, Bozzola E, Meazza C, Martinetti M,
Tinelli C, Corazza GR. Growth hormone deficiency and coeliac
disease: an unusual association?
Clin Endocrinol (Oxf). 2005; 62(3):372-5.

Braly, James and Hoggan, Ron.
Dangerous Grains: Why Gluten Cereal Grains May Be Hazardous
to Your Health. Book: 2002. Pub: Penguin Putnam Inc. NY. USA.

Collin P, Reunala T, Pukkala E, et al.
Coeliac disease – associated disorders and survival.
Gut 1994; 35: 1215-1218.

Collin P, Maki M.
Associated disorders in coeliac disease: clinical aspects.
Scand J Gastroenterol 1994; 29: 769-775.

Cooke WT, Thomas-Smith W.
Neurological disorders associated with adult coeliac disease.
Brain 1966; 89: 683-722

Corazza GR, Andreani ML, Venuro N, et al.
Celiac disease and alopecia areata: report of a new association.
Gastroenterology 1995; 109: 1333-1337.

Corvaglia L, Catamo R, Pepe G, Lazzari R, Corvaglia E.
Depression in adult untreated celiac subjects: diagnosis by the
pediatrician. Am J Gastroenterol. 1999; 94(3):839-43.

Cronin CC, Jackson LM, Feighery C, et al.
Coeliac disease and epilepsy.
QJM 1998; 91: 303-308.

Cuomo A, Romano M, Rocco A, et al.
Reflux oesophagitis in adult coeliac disease: beneficial effects of a
gluten free diet Gut 2003; 52: 514-517.

De Sanctis A, Addolorato G, Romito A, et al.
Schizophrenic symptoms and SPECT abnormalities in a coeliac
patient: regression after a gluten-free diet.
J Intern Med 1997; 242: 421-423.

Dicke WK, Weijers HA, Van De Kamer JH.
Coeliac disease II: the presence in wheat of a factor having a
deleterious effect in cases of coeliac disease.
Acta Paediatrica 1953; 42: 34-42.

Dohan FC. Cereals and Schizophrenia: Data and hypothesis.
Acta Psychiatr. Scand 1966 ; 42:125-42

Dohan FC.
More on Celiac Disease as a model for schizophrenia.
Biol. Psychiatry 1983; 18:561-4.

Duggan J M Coeliac disease: the great imitator
MJA 2004; 180 (10): 524-526.

Fasano, A., Not T, Wang W, Uzzau S, Berti I, Tommasini A, Goldblum SE. Zonulin, a newly discovered modulator of intestinal permeability, and its expression in coeliac disease.
Lancet 2000, 355: 1518-1519.

Fasano A, Not T, Wang W, Uzzau S, Berti I, Tommasini A, Goldblum SE. Zonulin, a newly discovered modulator of intestinal permeability, and its expression in coeliac disease.
Lancet. 2000; 355(9214):1518-9.

Fasano A. Regulation of intercellular tight junctions by zonula occludens toxin and its eukaryotic analogue zonulin (review).
Ann N Y Acad Sci. 2000; 915:214-22.

Fasano A.
Celiac disease – how to handle a clinical chameleon.
N Engl J Med 2003; 348: 2568-2570.

Fasano A, Berti I, Gerarduzzi T.
Prevalence of celiac disease in at-risk and not-at-risk groups in the United States. Arch Intern Med 2003; 163: 286-292.

Federico G, Favilli T, Cinquanta L, Ughi C, Saggese G.
Effect of celiac disease and gluten-free diet on growth hormone-binding protein, insulin-like growth factor-I, and insulin-like growth factor-binding proteins.
Horm Res. 1997;48(3):108-14.

Fine KD.
Small Bowel Enteropathy in Patients with Microscopic Colitis: Is It Gluten-Sensitive? J Clin Gastroenterol 2001;32:193-195.

Fois A, Vascotto M, Di Bartolo RM, Di Marco V.
Celiac disease and epilepsy in pediatric patients.
Childs Nerv Syst. 1994; 10(7):450-4.

Fonager K, Sorensen HT, Norgard B, Thulstrup AM.
Cardiomyopathy in Danish patients with coeliac disease.
Lancet 1999; 354: 1561.

Ford RPK, Menzies IS, Phillips AD, WalkerSmith JA, Turner
MW. Intestinal sugar permeability : relationship to diarrhoeal
disease and small bowel morphology.
J Pediatr Gastro Nutr. 1985; 4: 568-574.

Gale L, Wimalaratna H, Brotodiharjo A, Duggan JM.
Down syndrome is strongly associated with coeliac disease.
Gut 1997; 40: 492-496.

Gasparrini A, Torre ES, Trivellini C, et al.
Recurrent spontaneous abortion and intrauterine fetal growth
retardation as symptoms of coeliac disease.
Lancet 2000; 356: 399-400.

Gee S.
On the coeliac affection.
St Bartholomew's Hospital reports 1888; 24: 17-20.

Gershon, Michael D.
The Second Brain: a groundbreaking new understanding of nerv-
ous disorders of the stomach and intestine.
(Your gut has a mind of its own)
Book 1998. Pub HarperCollins, NY, USA.

Gobbi G.
Coeliac disease, epilepsy and cerebral calcifications.
Brain Dev. 2005; 27(3):189-200.

Green PHR, Jabri B.
Coeliac disease.
Lancet 2003; 362: 383-391.

Hadjivassiliou M, Gibson A, Davies-Jones GAB, Lobo A, Stephenson T J, Milford-Ward A. Is cryptic gluten sensitivity an important cause of neurological illness?
Lancet 1996; 347: 369-371.

Hadjivassiliou M, Gibson A, Grünewald RA, Davies-Jones GAB, Chattopadhyay AK, Kandler RH, et al. Idiopathic ataxia of late onset: gluten sensitivity is part of the answer.
J Neurol Neurosurg Psychiatry 1997; 63: 267.

Hadjivassiliou M, Chattopadhyay AK, Davies-Jones GAB, Gibson A, Grünewald RA, Lobo AJ.
Neuromuscular disorder as a presenting feature of coeliac disease.
J Neurol Neurosurg Psychiatry 1997; 63: 770-775.

Hadjivassiliou M, Grünewald RA, Chattopadhyay AK, Davies-Jones GAB, Gibson A, Jarratt JA, et al.
Clinical, radiological, neurophysiological and neuropathological characteristics of gluten ataxia. Lancet 1998; 352: 1582-1585.

Hadjivassiliou M, Boscolo S, Davies-Jones GA, Grunewald RA, Not T, Sanders DS, Simpson JE, Tongiorgi E, Williamson CA, Woodroofe NM. The humoral response in the pathogenesis of gluten ataxia. Neurology. 2002;58:1221-6.

Hadjivassiliou M, Grunewald RI, Sharrack B, et al.
Gluten ataxia in perspective: epidemiology, genetic susceptibility and clinical characteristics. Brain 2003; 126: 685-691.

Hoffenberg EJ, Emery LM, Barriga KJ, Bao F, Taylor J, Eisenbarth GS, Haas JE, Sokol RJ, Taki I, Norris JM, Rewers M. Clinical features of children with screening-identified evidence of celiac disease. Pediatrics. 2004; 113(5):1254-9.

Hoffman, Ronald. Tired All the Time: How to Regain Your Lost Energy. Book 1993: Pub Poseidon Press.

Holmes GK, Prior P, Lane MR, et al.
Malignancy in coeliac disease – effect of a gluten free diet.
Gut 1989; 30: 333-338.

Holmes GKT. Non-malignant complications of coeliac disease.
Acta Paediatr Suppl 1996; 412: 68-75.

Illingworth, Ronald S. The normal child: some problems of early years and their treatment.
Book. 1991. Pub. Churchill Livingston. UK.

Korn, Danna.
Wheat free, worry-free. The art of happy, healthy gluten-free living. Book. 2002. Pub: Hay House Inc. CA. USA

Knivsberg A-M, Reichelt K, Holin T, Nodland M.
A randomised controlled trial of dietary intervention in autistic syndromes. Nutritional Neuroscience 2002;5:251-261.

Kreek MJ, Schaefer RA, Hahn EF, Fishman J.
Naloxone, a specific opioid antagonist, reverses chronic idiopathic constipation. Lancet. 1983; 1(8319):261-2.

Lindh E, Ljunghall S, Larsson K, Lavo B.
Screening for antibodies against gliadin in patients with osteoporosis. J Intern Med 1992; 231: 403-406.

Lo W, Sano K, Lebwohl B, et al. Changing presentation of adult celiac disease. Dig Dis Sci 2003; 48: 395-398.

Lowell, Jax Peters. Against the grain.
Book. 1995. Pub: Henry Holt Co. USA.

Lubrano E, Ciacci C, Ames PR, et al.
The arthritis of coeliac disease: prevalence and pattern in 200
patients. Br J Rheumatol 1996; 35: 1314-1318.

Maki M, Collin P. Coeliac disease.
Lancet 1997; 349: 1755-1759.

Marks J, Shuster S, Watson AJ.
Small bowel changes in dermatitis herpetiformis.
Lancet 1966; ii: 1280-1282.

Mills PR, Brown IL, Ojetti V, Sanchez JA, Guerriero C, et al.
High prevalence of celiac disease in psoriasis.
Gastroenterology 2003; Suppl 1: A656.

Maria Teresa Pellecchia, Rossana Scala, Alessandro Filla,
Giuseppe De Michele, Carolina Ciacci, Paolo Baronea.
Idiopathic cerebellar ataxia associated with celiac disease: lack of
distinctive neurological features
J Neurol Neurosurg Psychiatry 1999;66:32-35

Marsh MN.
The natural history of gluten sensitivity: defining, refining and re-
defining. *Q J Med* 1995; 85: 9-13.

Marti T, Molberg O, Li Q, Gray GM, Khosla C, Sollid LM.
Prolyl Endopeptidase Mediated Destruction of T Cell Epitopes in
whole Gluten - Chemical and Immunological Characterization.
J Pharmacol Exp Ther. 2005 Jan;312(1):19-26. Epub 2004 Sep 9.

Mercola, Joseph. The no-grain diet.
Book, 2005. Pub Hodder and Stoughton. USA.

Parnell NDJ, Ciclitra PJ. Review article: coeliac disease and its
management. Aliment Pharmacol Ther 1999; 13: 1-13.

Ranua J, Luoma K, Auvinen A, Maki M, Haapala AM, Peltola J, Raitanen J, Isojarvi J. Celiac disease-related antibodies in an epilepsy cohort and matched reference population. Epilepsy Behav. 2005; 6(3):388-92.

Sanders DS, Carter MJ, Hurlstone DP, et al.
Association of adult coeliac disease with irritable bowel syndrome: a case-control study in patients fulfilling ROME II criteria referred to secondary care. Lancet 2001; 358: 1504-1508.

Sjoberg K, Eriksson KF, Bredberg A, et al.
Screening for coeliac disease in adult insulin-dependent diabetes mellitus. J Intern Med 1998; 243: 133-140.

Sher K, Mayberry J.
Female fertility, obstetric and gynaecological history in coeliac disease: a case control study.
Gastroenterology 1994; 55: 243-246.

Sher KS, Jayanthi V, Probert CSJ, et al.
Infertility, obstetric and gynaecological problems in coeliac disease.
Dig Dis 1994; 12: 186-190.

Smith, Melissa Diane. Going Against The Grain: How reducing and avoiding grains can revitalize your health.
Book:2002. Pub. Contemporary Books. McGraw-Hill N.Y.

Troncone R, Greco L, Mayer M, Paparo F, Caputo N, Micillo M.
Latent and potential coeliac disease.
Acta Paediatr 1996; 412 (suppl): 10-14.

Tursi A.
Gastrointestinal motility disturbances in celiac disease.
J Clin Gastroenterol 2004; 38: (8):642-5.

Usai P.
Adult coeliac disease is frequently associated with sacroiliitis.
Dig Dis Sci 1995; 40: 1906-1908.

Usai P, Usai Satta P, Lai M, Corda MG, Piras E, Calcara C, Boy MF, Morelli A, Balestrieri A, Bassotti G.
Autonomic dysfunction and upper digestive functional disorders in untreated adult coeliac disease.
Eur J Clin Invest 1997;27:1009-1015.

Visakorpi, 1970 Visakorpi JK, Kuitunen P, Savilahti E.
Frequency and nature of relapses in children suffering from the malabsorption syndrome with gluten intolerance.
Acta Paediatr Scand. 1970; 59(5):481-6.

Vogelsang H, Oberhuber G, Wyatt J.
Lymphocytic gastritis and gastric permeability in patients with celiac disease.
Gastroenterology 1996; 111: 73-77.

Weinstein WM.
Latent celiac sprue.
Gastroenterology 1974; 66: 489-493.

Wilkinson G.
Idiopathic chronic ulcerative enteritis.
QJM 1980; 49: 133-149.

Wills AJ.
The neurology and neuropathology of coeliac disease.
Neuropathol Appl Neurobiol. 2000; 26(6):493-6.

Zelnik N, Pacht A, Obeid R, Lerner A.
Range of neurologic disorders in patients with celiac disease.
Pediatrics. 2004; 113(6):1672-6.

Gluten-free recipes for you – free

We would like to give you some recipes.
These are free for you. Just go to the website
www.doctorgluten.com
All you have to do is put in your user name
and password. Then you can get your free
recipes and much more information.

Go to **www.doctorgluten.com**

Your User name: **gluten**
Your Password: **free**

Then you can get your free recipes

☐The Energy Effect? Your Questions Answered

Dr Rodney Ford, nutritional and energy expert, teaches you how to
live each day with High Energy. He shows you how to use the
combination of your body, brain and spirit to create – The Energy
Effect. Do you find that you lack time or energy to do all that you
want? Do you want feel energized so you can keep on going – and
going – to the end of your day? The Energy Effect gives you complete
answers on how to create more energy in your life.

ISBN 0-473-10259-5 (192 pages)   (NZ$34.95 Aus$34.95 US$19.95)

☐Going Gluten-Free: How to Get Started

"Overwhelm" is often the first emotion felt when you are confronted by
the prospect of a gluten-free diet. Find out how you can get started.
Step1– Get ready: Identify if you really are gluten-sensitive. Check out
your symptoms and blood tests. Step 2 – Get set up: Find out all
about gluten. Use our shopping list to help you work out what you can
eat and what you should avoid. Step 3 – Go gluten-free: Follow the
recipes and eating ideas. Gluten-free can be a great experience.

ISBN 0-473-10491-1 (64 pages)   (NZ$14.95 Aus$14.95 US$9.95)

See our other books

☐Are You Gluten-Sensitive? Your Questions Answered

This book is based on the questions that I am so frequently asked by my patients. I answer their questions in detail and put them into the clinical context. There is lots of confusion about the diagnosis and management of people who are gluten-sensitive. This book has been written to clarify this muddle. It is full of practical information.

ISBN 0-476-00917-0 (192 pages)   (NZ$34.95 Aus$34.95 US$19.95)

☐The gluten-free lunch book

What can I have for lunch? That is our most often asked question. Easy and yummy lunches make all the difference if you are trying to stay gluten-free. We have brought together the best lunch ideas so that you never have to worry about lunch again. Simple and delicious gluten-free lunch box ideas for you and your family. Follow these recipes and eating ideas for a great gluten-free experience.

ISBN 0-473-10498-9 (64 pages)   (NZ$14.95 Aus$14.95 US$9.95)

☐The book for the **Sick, Tired & Grumpy** (Gluten-free kids)

Over 50 people tell their amazing stories. A cure for so many people who feel sick, tired or grumpy. These personal accounts are very moving with a raw honesty that hits home. If you want to feel well and full of energy again – then this book is for you. These children and parents tell about their low energy, their irritability and troublesome symptoms before they discovered their gluten-sensitivity. You then hear how going gluten-free has changed their lives. This might be just the answer you are looking for.

ISBN 0-473-10079-7 (192 pages)   (NZ$34.95 Aus$34.95 US$19.95)

☐Full of it! The shocking truth about gluten

An alarming fact is that gluten can damage your brain. Have you ever wondered why you crave for another hunk of bread? If a food that you ate was slowly eroding the function and the ability of your brain, then would you want to know what that food was? It is gluten! Gluten is linked to ataxia, migraine, ADHD, autism, depression, epilepsy, mood and psychiatric disorders.   Gluten also can disrupt your brain's regulation of your gut – causing mayhem in your bowel.   Gluten-sensitivity is a brain disease! Read the evidence for yourself.

ISBN 0-473-10407-5 (192 pages)   (NZ$34.95 Aus$34.95 US$19.95)

Available from our website: www.doctorgluten.com

❑**Are You Gluten-Sensitive? Your Questions Answered**

❑**Going Gluten-Free: How to Get Started**

❑**The Gluten-Free Lunch Book**

❑**The book for the Sick, Tired & Grumpy**

❑**Full of it! The shocking truth about gluten**

❑**The Energy Effect? Your Questions Answered**

(Please indicate the number of each book that you want to order. Prices stated on previous page)

Please add postage & handling: 1 book $7.00, 2 books $12, 3 or 4 books $15

(Prices for postage and handling to be paid in the currency of purchase)

Order for:

Name: _____

Postal address: _____

_____

Phone: _____ Fax: _____

Email: _____@ _____

Number of books required: _____ Currency _____

Cost of books $ _____ Postage $ _____ Total $_____

Method of payment:

Cheque ❑   Visa ❑   MasterCard ❑   (please tick)

Cardholder's name: _____

Credit card number : _____

Signature: _____ Expiry date: _____/_____

Please make your cheque payable to:

Doctor Gluten, PO Box 25-360, Christchurch, New Zealand.

Fax orders: +64 3 3770596

Email orders: orders@doctorgluten.com

Web orders: www.doctorgluten.com

(Please allow 21 days for postal delivery)